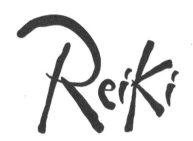

THE TRUE STORY

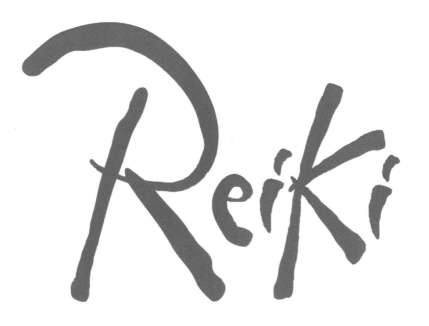

THE TRUE STORY

An Exploration of Usui Reiki

DON BECKETT

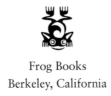

Frog Books
Berkeley, California

Published by Frog Books, an imprint of North Atlantic Books
Berkeley, California

Cover and book design by Brad Greene
Printed in the United States of America

Reiki: The True Story—An Exploration of Usui Reiki is sponsored and published by the Society for the Study of Native Arts and Sciences (dba North Atlantic Books), an educational nonprofit based in Berkeley, California, that collaborates with partners to develop cross-cultural perspectives, nurture holistic views of art, science, the humanities, and healing, and seed personal and global transformation by publishing work on the relationship of body, spirit, and nature.

North Atlantic Books' publications are available through most bookstores. For further information, visit our website at www.northatlanticbooks.com or call 800-733-3000.

Library of Congress Cataloging-in-Publication Data

Beckett, Don, 1953–
    Reiki, the true story : an exploration of Usui reiki / Don Beckett.
        p. cm.
    Includes bibliographical references and index.
    ISBN 978-1-58394-267-3
    1. Reiki (Healing system) 2. Spiritual healing. I. Title.
    RZ403.R45B43 2008
    615.8'51—dc22

                                                            2008026745

3 4 5 6 7 8 9 SHERIDAN 21 20 19 18 17

North Atlantic Books is committed to the protection of our environment. We partner with FSC-certified printers using soy-based inks and print on recycled paper whenever possible.

To Mikao Usui and Mokichi Okada

I'm also eternally grateful to:

- Oxana Alekseeva, without whose motivation this project would not have been born;

- the island of Kaua'i (where the first incarnation of this book was written), without whose introspective and focused energy, as well as inspiration, the writing, if completed at all, would certainly have taken longer and been of lesser quality;

- Donna Lee, without whose generous aloha spirit I would not have had a place to live and write;

- my parents, Don and Dorothy, most of all, without whose life-long aid and support and guidance I would not have been here to write anything!

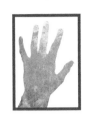

Contents

I feel much honored to have been involved in the very first print edition of Don Beckett's Reiki book. That was in 2006 and it was a Turkish translation. I had read the original e-book more than a year before and was delighted by Beckett's approach to Reiki, as well as the great scope of information he presented. It was, and is more so with this revised and expanded edition, an invaluable source for everyone involved in or just now attracted to Reiki.

I had wanted to share this gift with the people of my country. It took me more than a year to find a publisher interested in a new Reiki book. Yes, we had more than enough Reiki books in print then, written by Turkish and foreign authors. Yet what we had on the shelves were more or less repetitions of the same outdated story or some quick-fix cure-all guides, in tune with and responding to mass consciousness. Nothing like the book you are holding now. After many communications with various publishers, just when I was about to give up the idea, unexpected synchronicities smoothed out the way to the Turkish edition. I still wonder why Beckett's book appeared in print for the first time in a country exactly at the other end of the world from where he was then living: Hawai'i and Turkey have a twelve-hour time difference!

What makes this book an invaluable source for everyone who wants to get a closer look at Reiki is the extensive and detailed picture of Reiki's history. It is "The True Story," to the extent of our current knowledge: a compilation of information transmitted by people who personally knew Mikao Usui. In addition to this detailed picture, Don Beckett presents three levels of training, as learned by students of Usui himself. Based on his own seventeen years of experience in Reiki, Beckett also provides enlightening insights on such things as: What Really Happens in a Reiki Empowerment? What is True Healing? Kotodama Pronunciation and How to Make the Sounds—to name a few.

But what especially makes this book unique is his emphasis on Reiki being a way to get to know your Self. Your real Self. "I can't overemphasize that Reiki is about connecting to your true Self, to your innermost knowledge," says Don Beckett. It is one of the many ways to Self-realization, to remembering and reactivating your Divine connection. Reiki attunements or empowerments are only about self-empowerment. And isn't self-empowerment actually the remembrance of your inherent connection to All That Is? What can empower you more than this connectedness? What else can set you free from the web of illusions? Thus Beckett writes: "One of the great things about Reiki is that it encourages personal freedom." Yes, self-empowerment is the road to freedom.

With its emphasis on personal freedom, this book is not a *follow-me, I'll safely and quickly guide you through* book. "Any techniques you learn from someone else are only starting points—and even the techniques you develop for yourself are merely tools. It's important not to invest them with powers they don't actually possess." Techniques and guidelines are not meant to dominate us; "the very nature of Reiki is to engender diversity and variety!"

So, read the book, choose any points that resonate with you, shuffle and restructure them, and develop your own guidebook. Take any ideas you like, and explore and expand them according to your taste. You can do this again and again. Release any ideas that do not serve you anymore and choose others. For Reiki, like other paths to Self-realization, is a continual process, a never-ending journey towards unlimited horizons, where "change" and "expansion" are the keywords.

When I got my first- and second-degree Reiki attunements, in 1995 and 1996, all I had learned about the origins of Reiki was that brief Takata version: Mikao Usui, a Japanese Christian priest, dedicates his life to discovering the secret of how Jesus healed the sick. His quest and travels end on Mount Kurama, where, after a twenty-one-day fast, he is hit by some bright light and the Reiki symbols are showered upon him. The addenda to this brief story were not so very brief, though. The importance of "energy exchange" was deliberately and lengthily covered and the sacredness and secrecy of the Reiki symbols were duly emphasized.

Those were the days when different and controversial versions of Reiki history were being disclosed one after the other, shattering the Takata version; and the first book cracking the taboo on Reiki symbols had only recently appeared in print. The dominance of The Reiki Alliance was being challenged by the many independent Reiki teachers, or "Masters." Then came all those Reikis with various different names. As for me, I was still happy with my Usui Shiki Ryoho. Enjoying the miracles through Reiki was enough for me then. The upheaval in the Reiki community didn't interest me much.

Eight years later, I decided to be a Reiki teacher. I got my third-degree attunement and my certificate as a Reiki teacher. If you want to learn any subject, better attempt to teach it. When you are there to teach, you cannot teach just by transmitting others' experiences and interpretations; you have to internalize all knowledge about your subject. So, being a Reiki teacher pushed me forward to a new understanding of Reiki. I saw that I hadn't really known what Reiki was about. Yes, I had memorized that it was "universal life energy." But what did that really mean? I had witnessed miraculous healings. But what did "healing" mean? Maybe it was about remembering that we didn't need any "healings," that we were already perfect as we were. . . . What was the true essence of Reiki? What made it unique, or was it only its name that was unique? None of my Reiki teachers' explanations resonated with me. Neither did any of the books I had read on Reiki. I learned best through my own experiences and from feedback I got from my patients. And I kept on questioning, because each new answer brought forward a new question.

It was during those days that I got to know Don Beckett. His Reiju from the other end of the world had been a great energetic experience for me. I remember that then the MD aspect of me had thought my blood pressure was up: I was going around like a steam engine, with rhythmic puffs in my ears! Then he very generously sent me his Shoden (first-level Reiki) training manual. Exchanging thoughts and ideas by email got more frequent in time. I was happy that at last I could find a teacher whose approach to Reiki did much resonate with mine. Much later, I had the honor to get to know Don in person. What I saw was a very gentle and sensitive nature, an inherent respect for all forms of life, combined with intellectual acuity and curiosity. His extremely simple lifestyle was keeping him way out of the hubbub of mass consciousness. Getting to know him in person made me see why his book was unique: He wouldn't settle for clichés or stereotypical explanations. He wouldn't be at ease unless he delved deeply enough and reached answers that he felt were satisfactory—at least until new questions arose from the yet newer understanding.

"The human body is a hologram of All That Is." Thus, it encompasses all the elements, as well as all knowledge. This understanding shapes Beckett's Reiki practice. His "You Are The Universe!" self-healing method is a reflection of such an awareness. He directs the energy to the whole universe while he is "giving" himself Reiki. He does not "send" Reiki distantly; he reaches in and out to Unity, where there is no past or future, far or near.

He believes that empowerment is a matter of conscious awareness. "Possibly what gives greatest effectiveness and empowers us the most is accurate understanding: having a concept that aligns with reality." Thus, his insistent emphasis on the Reiki Concepts. "The Reiki Concepts make Reiki a way of life, not just a transmission of healing energy to be turned on and off." When we incorporate these Concepts into our lives "from morning to night," it will affect "what kind of energy we generate ourselves, all the time. This is where the Concepts prove to be so important." The energy we generate ourselves can be such that "there comes a time when Reiki empowerment can be given merely by intent, with no procedure at all." And I believe that, as it was with Mikao Usui, there comes a time when we can even move beyond intent—to where our mere presence will be empowering to those seeking self-empowerment, Self-realization.

Beckett discusses many controversial issues, such as the Reiki symbols ("Reiki symbols are not Reiki. It's much better to get beyond the symbols, to the Source"), Reiki Masters ("Reiki Mastery is really mastery of ourselves"), the much-emphasized "energetic exchange" issue, and "healing attunements." He consistently grounds his arguments in the original Usui teachings and adds his personal interpretation. The information he provides on kotodama and how they are used in Reiki is not widely cited in other Reiki sources, and sounds like an appealing and easy practice, worth a try.

As humanity is now approaching the shift of the ages, we are releasing many of the concepts and techniques that resonate with the old. And if we are to welcome the shift, we have to rely on none other than our own inner guidance. "It's important to keep moving forward with the stream of our intuition as it leads us always to new and better things," says Don Beckett. Throughout the vast spectrum of information in this book, the recurrent theme is trusting your intuition and getting in touch with your innermost knowledge. Very appropriately so, because intuition and knowingness are messages from your real Self, and because Reiki is only about you, yourself.

Reiki is not about rules; it is you who write your own rules. Reiki is not about sacred and secret symbols, either. You yourself are sacred and you are here to remember that secret. Reiki is here to help you remember. But, as with other paths towards such a realization, remembrance through Reiki has been blocked or complicated for many. A net of rules and symbols has entrapped the understanding and the practice of Reiki, almost to the verge of suffocation. *Reiki: The True Story* is a book that delivers a much-needed breath of fresh air, clearing the path to remembrance.

—Zeyneb Umit Belbez

Reiki Teacher, MD (board-certified in Internal Medicine),
and PhD student in History of Medicine and Medical Ethics

Author's Note to the 2009 Edition

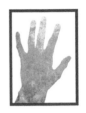

This work was initially undertaken in late 2002, intended for publication in Russia. The twists and turns of life delayed that publication until 2007, by which time the work had appeared as an e-book (seven editions, 2005–2006) and as a printed edition in Turkish (2006).

This book, the one you're holding now, incorporates updated material from the "outside" world, along with changes in my personal viewpoint, perception, and understanding since the earlier incarnations of the work.

—db

Mesa, Arizona
June 2008

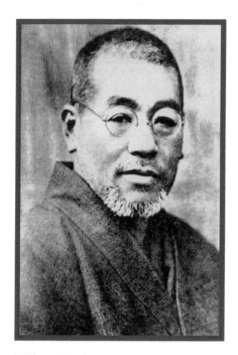

Mikao Usui
Image courtesy Matthieu Briand
(www.reikimatt.com/)

Today only
Anger not
Worry not
Do your work with appreciation
Be kind to people

(Translation of Usui Concepts, courtesy Dave King)

Acknowledgments

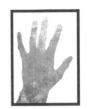

I'm grateful to the following, for material and inspiration that have gone into this book:

Phil Morgan, my first Reiki teacher, for giving me a good start on the path;

Deb Frank, my next Reiki teacher, whose great generosity allowed me to become a Reiki "Master" at just the right time to receive training and priceless inspiration from ...

Hiroshi Doi-sensei, at the very first Usui Reiki Ryoho International conference, arranged by ...

Rick Rivard, Tom Rigler, and Andrew Bowling;

Arjava Petter and Chetna Kobayashi, for additional training and inspiration;

Karen Smith;

Adonea and Light;

and, most of all, teachings of early students of Mikao Usui, and of students of those students—via Dave King and Melissa Riggall (a.k.a. Shen-Lissa), and Chris Marsh via Taggart King.

Great thanks to Rev. Michael Daniel Neary, for healing and inspiration, and for expanding my understanding of Johrei.

Also ...

Mana Hirose, for Japanese-English translations;

Michael Ash and Mio, for illustration photos and calligraphy.

Additional thanks to the following, for their generous gifts of healing and enlightenment:

Angela Anchor

Zeyneb Belbez

Akram Khan

Nina Dunn

Helene Eager

Nichijo Fumon

Jo Hammel

Rebecca Hardcastle

the johreiki.net Healing Circle

Fara Kaufman

Michael Daniel Neary

Roger Orcutt

Julie Parry

Dragan Pavlovic

Phillip & Deborah

Thanks to Nina, for finding North Atlantic Books.

Thanks to Pearleen, for getting the crucial pictures here, just in time!

Thanks to Kathy Glass, for editing (and, in addition to removing my excessive commas and semicolons and exclamation marks, asking questions that brought forth some good answers).

And special thanks to James Deacon (www.aetw.org) for providing the translation of the Usui Memorial inscription. In return, I told him I would mention one of his favorite charities:

The Dian Fossey Gorilla Fund International (www.gorillafund.org/)

800 Cherokee Ave., SE, Atlanta, Georgia 30315-1440, U.S.A.

Introduction

Rei-ki. The word, often used by spiritual healers in Japan since at least the 1860s, came from China (where it's pronounced *Ling-chi*). Most people today use it to refer to a method of healing with subtle energy. There are many Reiki methods, many styles and variations, being taught today. To the best of my knowledge, all of them owe their existence to a method created in the early 1900s by Mikao Usui. According to students who were taught by Usui himself, his original teachings were aimed at Self-realization, not directly at the healing of others; and he called them simply "a method to achieve personal perfection."

By the time of Usui's passing in 1926, several versions of his method were being taught in Japan. These were directed more to the healing of others than to one's own spiritual awakening. Shortly after the passing of Usui, a memorial society—the Usui Reiki Ryoho Gakkai (Usui Reiki Healing Method Society)—was created in his honor.

In 1938, the world outside Japan got its first taste of what has come to be known as Reiki. A Japanese-American woman named Hawayo Takata, who had been healed through Reiki in Japan (at the clinic of one of Mikao Usui's final students), returned to her home in Hawai'i and was later certified there to teach her own version of Reiki. Takata herself did not initiate any Reiki teachers for almost forty years—until 1976. From that time on, the practice of Reiki has spread around the world, mushrooming especially in recent years.

Until the mid-1990s, the Takata version of Reiki, and its derivatives, made up the sum of Reiki knowledge in the world outside Japan. Many of us who were taught the Takata version felt something "not quite right" about it—the history of Reiki as given, and . . . it just felt that something was *missing*.

Then a Canadian Reiki teacher, Dave King,[1] began discovering some illuminating things. He and a colleague, Melissa Riggall (later known as Shen-Lissa), had in fact learned some original Usui teachings, as a form of Chi-gung, way back in 1971. On a visit to Morocco, they had been taught by a man who had learned from a close friend and student of Usui himself. These teachings were nothing like what we know as Usui Reiki. When Dave and Melissa got involved in Reiki and began making trips to Japan (in the 1990s), they started meeting numerous people with connections to Usui. Some had been students of Usui himself; some were students of Usui's students; at least one had learned both Usui's original method for spiritual awakening and the first "healing" method that had grown out of it.

Also in the '90s, Frank Arjava Petter[2] and his wife, Chetna Kobayashi, were living in Japan and researching the origin of Reiki. It was during this time that the gravesite memorial to Mikao Usui was introduced to the world at large.

In 1999, we were given the first presentation (outside Japan) of the Usui Reiki Ryoho Gakkai's view of Reiki.[3]

In the year 2000, an English Reiki teacher, Chris Marsh, was introduced to a student of Mikao Usui (a Buddhist nun, 106 years old at the time) in Japan. She began teaching him what she had learned from Usui; and, the following year, Chris was introduced to eleven more Usui students, all of them around a hundred years old.

These recent revelations from Japan have been, and continue to be, enormously helpful in putting together a more accurate picture of the origin and history of what is now called Usui Reiki.

Part Three of this book is titled "The Mystery," a translation of the Japanese word *shinpiden,* which is the name of the third degree in Usui Reiki.[4] However, the mysteries of Usui Reiki are not confined to Shinpiden; there are mysteries at every level. For instance, questions as basic as:

When did Mikao Usui begin teaching his method?

Did he call it Reiki or something else?

Did he give it a name at all?

Did he found the Usui Reiki Ryoho Gakkai, as its members claim, or was it begun after his death, by three naval officers among his students?

Is the legendary story of his Reiki empowerment on Mount Kurama in 1922 (as told by the Usui Gakkai) accurate or not?

There is lack of consensus in the Reiki world regarding the answers to these questions and many more. So much research has been done by numerous people, and yet—even now, with firsthand information from those who were taught by Usui himself in the early 1900s—there are still mysteries about Usui the man and the history of Usui Reiki. Different researchers tell different stories, and information is often unverifiable.

One thing we do know: With much disagreement, sometimes even hostilities, among various Reiki factions; with new brands of Reiki (some even trademarked) being created faster than flavors of ice cream; with attempts (successful in some cases) even to trademark the word

Reiki itself—the great news is that *Mikao Usui's gift to the world is alive and well and flourishing globally as never before!* The energy connection, the "extension cord" to universal Source energy that Usui provided for us all, is growing stronger by the day, growing to cover our beleaguered planet in a web of healing and empowerment, just now when we need it most, as we accelerate into what may be the greatest transformation in human history.

Part One

The Entrance (Shoden)

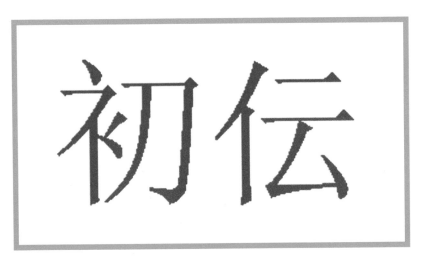

Kanji image courtesy Dave King

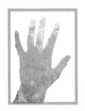

Chapter 1

Beginnings and History

What Is Reiki?

Reiki is a Japanese word, often translated as "universal life energy." It also means "soul force" or "spiritual power." In Japan the general term for life energy is *ki*, and Rei-ki is seen as the highest of seven energies responsible for life in the material universe (see "*Ki*, the Energy of Life" in Chapter 5). Being at the top of this hierarchy, Reiki is positioned at the meeting place of the physical and spiritual realms; it bridges the material world and the world of pure Spirit.

The Japanese *kanji* of Reiki has two parts:

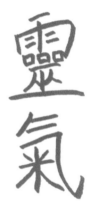

Rei	and	Ki

 The deliberate action of bringing "rain" (Heavenly power) down to Earth.

 The asterisk-like figure is "rice," the staple food of human life. The other lines are the aura of the rice.

If we look at each part as a separate word, *Rei* can be translated as "spirit" and *Ki* simply as "energy." We may think of Ki as our personal energy (sustained by eating the rice), and Rei-ki as the action of bringing down the energy of Heaven or the greater Universe (Rei) and uniting it with our personal Ki.[1] This brings "enlightenment," which is another translation of the word Reiki. Mr. Hiroshi Doi, a Japanese Reiki teacher and member of the Usui Reiki Ryoho Gakkai in Tokyo, says, "Reiki is wave of love!" I believe it is exactly that: a vibration of pure, unconditional love, which brings out the best in everything it touches. We can think of Reiki as the "extension cord" that connects us to Source energy, or the "program" that allows the integration of Source energy in the material world.

We Are All Healers

The human body is designed to maintain its own health constantly and automatically. It works day and night to nourish, revitalize, rebuild, relax, balance, and heal itself (despite our best efforts to sabotage all this!). In addition we have great powers of mind that can be consciously directed for healing. Our hands are particularly important in this. When our stomach hurts, when our head hurts, when we cut or bruise ourselves . . . we instinctively put our hands on the afflicted spot. It's natural for us to focus attention and healing through the hands.

As we already know, Reiki is an energy that allows and facilitates the integration of Source energy into the material world. And Reiki is part of our fundamental makeup. So, why are we not all transmitters of this healing energy? Ah, but we are—at least potentially! At birth and as babies we are very powerful transmitters of Source energy (which, I suspect, is what makes babies so attractive to most people). Then, as we settle increasingly into the lower vibrations of the physical world (a process accelerated and deepened by modern civilization and education), we "forget" our connection to Source. Our natural state of relaxation and ease becomes one of tension and dis-ease. The natural flow of energy becomes blocked and stagnant. Through Mikao Usui, we have been given an amazingly simple way of re-establishing our natural health and accelerating our spiritual awakening.

Usui Reiki Ryoho

It's generally agreed that Mikao Usui lived from August 15, 1865, to March 9, 1926, and that he had little formal education (though at least one Reiki scholar, Asunam Pope, believes that Usui received a Doctoral education in Literature[2]). He was obviously intelligent and a deep thinker, and he devoted his life to the study and practice of many things.

According to Taggart King, an English Reiki teacher and my primary source of the information coming from the Japanese students teaching Chris Marsh,[3] Usui entered a Tendai Buddhist monastery near Mount Kurama as a very young child. There he studied *Ki-ko* (the Japanese name for *Chi-gung*) and probably learned to do projection healings with it. He also attained the highest proficiency in a martial art called *Yagyu Ryu* (Samurai swordsmanship), as well as expertise in several other ancient martial arts.

In April 1922 Usui-sensei opened his first "seat of learning" in Harajuku, Tokyo.[4] He used a small manual, which had been created about 1920. It consisted of the Reiki Precepts, meditations, and *waka* ("native poems").[5] There were no hand positions for healing others.

Perhaps the timing of this move to Tokyo is the basis for the story that Usui founded the URR Gakkai in April 1922. The naval officers (who actually started the Gakkai) were Usui's final students. They had only several months of training with Usui before he passed away in 1926, and it's unclear how much they knew of Usui's history. They may have believed that the opening of this "seat of learning" in 1922 marked the birth of his method, and therefore chose that date for the legendary founding of the Usui Gakkai.

According to Taggart King:[6]

Usui Sensei was interested in a great many things and seems to have studied voraciously. There was a large University library in Kyoto, and Japanese sources believe that he would have done most of his research there, where sacred texts from all over the world would have been held. He studied traditional Chinese medicine and Western medicine, numerology and astrology, and psychic and clairvoyant development.

It is known that Usui travelled to China, America and Europe several times to learn and study Western ways, and this practice was encouraged in the Meiji era. Usui followed a number of professions: public servant, office worker, industrialist, reporter, politician's secretary, missionary, and supervisor of convicts. Usui was private secretary to Shimpei Goto, who was Secretary of the Railroad, Postmaster General, and Secretary of the Interior and State. The phrase 'politician's secretary' can be taken as a euphemism for 'bodyguard.' It is during his time in diplomatic service that he may have had the opportunity to travel to other countries.

Interested in spiritual things, Usui studied the major religions of the world. According to Hiroshi Doi, Usui-sensei was a Shinto priest for a time, and at other times belonged to various Buddhist sects. One researcher (Asunam Pope) believes that Usui had a life-changing conversion to Shingon Buddhism as a young man.[7] Some of Usui's living students, however (including a family relative), say that he was strictly a Tendai Buddhist throughout his life (and, for a time, a *Zaike*, a Tendai priest who lives in his own home, not in a temple).

The name used by Mikao Usui to describe what he taught was merely "a method to achieve personal perfection." Sometimes he called it just "my method." According to Andrew Bowling, Usui began teaching his method in a formalized way about 1912.[8]

Some of Usui's living students refer to his method as Usui-do (Usui Way);[9] some as Usui Teáte (Usui Hand-application). They were not all taught the same things or taught in the same way. Usui tailored his teaching to the abilities and interests of each individual, and naturally his own understanding evolved over time as well.

By the time of his passing in 1926, there were several versions of his method being taught in Japan. Even among those calling it Usui-do, there were variations in the teaching: Some learned it strictly as a method of self-awakening, with levels and ceremonial rites of passage modeled after the Judo system of Jigoro Kano; others learned it as primarily a spiritual path, but including some focus on healing and an "empowerment" procedure called Reiju.

At this writing, we have three main sources of information on these subjects: the URR Gakkai; Dave King's information from Japanese students; and Chris Marsh's information from Japanese students.

Our information from the URR Gakkai (Society) comes mostly through the story told on the memorial stone at Usui's gravesite, and via Hiroshi Doi (who is a member of the Gakkai). Both Mr. Doi and some translations of the inscription on the memorial stone refer to Usui's teachings as "Usui Reiki Ryoho" ("Usui Reiki Healing Method"). Some translate this as "Reiho," which they say is merely a shortened form of "Reiki Ryoho." Others translate "Reiho" as "Spirit Method" or "Spiritual Method."

Both Dave and Chris, however, confirm that neither Usui nor his immediate students called his teachings Usui Reiki Ryoho. They also point out that the URR Gakkai was not founded by Usui (as told on some translations of the memorial stone);[10] that it was started by one or more naval officers among his final students, after his passing. And Dave's information (from a Buddhist nun who was with Usui every day during the time in question) belies the legendary story of Usui's Reiki empowerment on Mount Kurama in March 1922.

The URR Gakkai version of the origin of Usui Reiki, as told on the gravestone and by Mr. Doi, is indeed at variance with the version coming from Usui's living students. At about age fifty, according to Mr. Doi, Usui's interest in finding the purpose of his life became all-consuming. Eventually he spent three years in Zen meditation, seeking enlightenment—and still it didn't come. At that point, it is said, his Zen master advised him to "try dying"—and in desperation he went to Mount Kurama, a favorite place of spiritual seekers, and began to fast, apparently determined either to die or to receive enlightenment.

Supposedly, on the morning of the twenty-first day, he experienced a cosmic Reiki empowerment of some kind, which led to the creation of his healing method. The story on his gravestone says he felt a "large Reiki" over his head on Mount Kurama. And, in a training manual presented to students by the URR Gakkai, Usui is quoted as saying that he "accidentally realized" he had been given healing power, when he "felt the air in a mysterious way during fasting."

The living students, via Chris Marsh and Taggart King, also mention Usui undergoing three years of Zen training and experiencing *satori* (a moment of sudden understanding) during a fast on Mount Kurama. Beyond that, the details of the two versions don't seem to mesh. The Gakkai version has Usui finishing his three years of Zen training in 1922, which is when the students' version has him starting it. They say the Kurama episode was one of five times that Usui performed The Lotus Repentance meditation; and the satori he received then was not the basis of his teachings. Rather, the teachings were based in his knowledge of Tendai Buddhist and Shinto practices, and he was teaching them years before this experience on Mount Kurama. Indeed, if the Zen training had begun in 1922, the subsequent meditation would have been in 1925, only the year before Usui's passing.

According to Dave King, Usui developed the Teáte version of his teachings from the Usui-do version; and neither Teáte nor Usui-do involved an energetic "empowerment" procedure. Then, in November 1925, Usui's *dojo* was more or less taken over by a group of naval officers led by a rear admiral named Ushida (a.k.a. Gyuda). A high entrance fee was levied on students then, and Usui's teachings were being presented by a close friend and student of Usui, Toshihiro Eguchi.[11]

By January 1926, a method called Usui Reiki Ryoho had appeared. This was a version of Usui Teáte, developed under the influence of Ushida, Eguchi, and Dr. Chujiro Hayashi (who, years later, would teach and certify Hawayo Takata). According to Dave's information from Usui's student Tenon-in,[12] the palm-healing methods were being taught in the dojo by Eguchi and Hayashi, not by Usui himself (though he observed the teaching)—Hayashi and Eguchi being the only students of Usui to have completed all the levels of Usui-do training.

Chris Marsh, on the other hand, has been taught by students of Usui who learned either Usui-do or Usui Teáte, and who say that receiving frequent energetic empowerments (through a procedure called *Reiju*) was an important part of the method. Usui himself is said to have given Reiju by intent alone, with no formal procedure. The Reiju procedure learned by Chris's teachers, they say, came from Tendai Buddhism. Also, according to them, Dr. Hayashi was *not* a student long enough to learn the complete teachings before Mikao Usui's passing. (Yes, there *are* mysteries in the world of Reiki!)

Dave King's information, via Tenon-in, is that the levels of Usui Reiki

Ryoho were named *Shoden, Okuden,* and *Shinpiden*—though each level may have had sub-levels. Originally, those at Shinpiden level were allowed to teach; later, in the Usui Gakkai, the level of *Shihan* (Teacher) was added, and each branch (location) of the Gakkai had only one Shihan.

Dr. Hayashi is said to have taught these four levels, after 1931. His famous student Hawayo Takata, who did not start initiating teachers until 1976, changed the number of levels back to three at that time.

Like his own teacher, Hayashi-sensei taught different things to different students. One of his renowned students, a Mr. Tatsumi, taught what he had learned as Usui-do; another, a Mrs. Yamaguchi, called her version Jikiden Reiki;[13] and Hayashi's most famous student, Hawayo Takata—the single person most responsible for the spread and the perception of Reiki globally—called her version Usui Shiki Ryoho (Usui-Style Healing Method).

Naturally, what I teach is my own version of all this. I've chosen to call it Usui Reiki Ryoho—though much of it is based on information from living students of Mikao Usui who themselves call it Usui-do. Also, my version is different than the version of Usui Reiki Ryoho taught by the Usui Gakkai. This book incorporates elements from various sources; I've done my best to identify those sources and also to present a fairly complete picture, historically.

Japan in the 1920s

During the 1920s Japan was awash with spiritual Societies and healing methods. Many of them contained the word *Rei* (as in Rei-ki), meaning Spirit. There was Dai Rei Do (a spiritual group, "Great Spirit Way") and Rei Shi Jitsu (a healing method), both started by Morihei Tanaka. There was even a Rei Ju Society, according to Fumio Ogawa, a member of the Usui Reiki Ryoho Gakkai.

In earlier years, Usui is said to have been involved with a group called Rei Jyutsu Kai ("Sublime Meeting of Souls"). They met at the base of Mount Kurama, north of Kyoto, and were renowned for clairvoyant and psychic development.

Another group, devoted to healing and spiritual purification, with allegedly some connection to Usui, would arise in the 1930s, using an energy that would later be called Johrei ("purifying spirit"). This was begun by a man named Mokichi Okada. In the 1920s he belonged to a spiritual group called Omoto Kyo, which had been started years earlier by a woman named Nao Deguchi. Her adopted son Onisaburo became its leader—and it's been said that both he and Okada were at some point students of Usui.[14] The Johrei method has many parallels to Reiki and, like Reiki, has spread around the world. Also like Usui Reiki, it has given birth to multiple offshoots.

Someone else who created his own spiritual/healing system was a close friend and prominent student of Usui, Toshihiro Eguchi, a school teacher. He learned the deepest secrets of Usui's method, and it's believed that it was he who taught Hayashi and the other founders of the Usui Gakkai how to give energetic empowerments. He also developed a method of his own, Te-no-hira Ryoji ("palm-of-the-hand healing"), and was allowed to teach it in Usui's dojo.

"A Method to Achieve Personal Perfection"

Mikao Usui was renowned as a healer, among other things. His healing abilities, and his great compassion for people, became especially well known after the great Kanto earthquake of 1923. It is said that his involvement in the healing of earthquake survivors led to his being given the honorary title of Doctor.

And yet healing *per se* was not the primary focus of his work.

People heard about him and came to ask for healing, and he gave healing—but he knew that the healing was only a secondary and inevitable effect of his "method to achieve personal perfection."

According to some of his students, when people came asking for healing, Usui would give them an energetic "empowerment" or "blessing." Called *Reiju* ("giving Spirit"), this was the first step in helping people to awaken to their own Source, to their own true identity. Reiju would be given each time the person returned; and, little by little, those who were interested would be instructed in Usui's method.

What was meant by "achieving personal perfection" was no less than Self-realization—the realization and manifesting of one's true spiritual identity. This is the integration of Universal Spirit *(Rei)* and personal energy *(ki)*, to bring enlightenment *(Rei-ki)*.

According to the stone at his grave, more than two thousand students received Usui's teachings in his last four years[15]—and now we know that he had been teaching his method much longer than that. After Usui's passing, Dr. Hayashi took upon himself the role of "successor"—which, after his own passing in 1940, was taken by his student Hawayo Takata.

Hiroshi Doi has said that Usui did not appoint or endorse anyone as his successor or lineage bearer (and it's clear that many students had been authorized to teach Usui's method, before his passing). Dave King (in *O-Sensei: A View of Mikao Usui*) says that Dr. Hayashi was indeed chosen by Usui to be his successor; and he confirms that Usui very deliberately did not allow his teachings to become the property of his family, or of any particular group. That would have been a customary thing to do, but Mikao Usui was determined to keep his method available to everyone.

Mariko's Memories

In 1996, Melissa Riggall met two Tendai Buddhist nuns in Nara, Japan: Yuri and Mariko (a.k.a. Tenon-in). They were with Mikao Usui from 1920 until his passing in 1926. Mariko was born in 1897. The following excerpts are from Mariko's story, as recorded in Melissa's diary:[16]

> Yuri and I met Usui-sama (O-Sensei) in 1920 on Hiei-zan[17] and soon after that we began working with him in a subdivision in the northwest of Kyoto. Later in the year we were joined by three more Tendai sisters. Usui had been developing a system of spiritual practices that made use of traditional values in those days of change in our country.

Mariko's description of Toshihiro Eguchi:

> On several occasions a very active man named Eguchi-sama appeared with bundles of cash. They spent hours together with Usui demonstrating his ideas while we had to make endless pots of tea and clean up.

Her description of March 1922 *(the month when Usui is supposed to have been fasting for twenty-one days on Mount Kurama, receiving his cosmic Reiki awakening)*:

> On March 3 we made one final trip to Hiei-zan and set off for Tokyo on the Nakasendo. We made many stops on the way and often walked between the villages. We arrived in Tokyo at the end of March.

And later:

> In early April O-Sensei found a small room in Harajuku.[18] Then came the earthquake of 1923. We all helped with the injured and the lost ones. Usui moved to a new room and at last had a separate place in which to sleep. Occasionally O-Sensei went out to work in the City.

Eguchi returned in 1923 with his own palm healing system that used parts of O-Sensei's work. It was almost a religion and part of this system was a ceremony that Eguchi had obtained from a friend named Nishida in which a form of blessing was offered to each *doka* [student]. This displeased Usui a great deal[19] but eventually Eguchi was permitted to come and teach at Usui's centre twice a week. Eguchi also had a small book printed which talked about healing methods and different techniques.

Mariko's memory of Dr. Hayashi's first appearance at the dojo:

In 1925 a group of high ranked naval officers arrived to learn the system. In May a commander named Hayashi arrived. He was always smiling at me and seemed to listen to what Usui had to say. Then in November two navy rear admirals appeared who were always complaining and demanding more information. The boss-man was called Gyuda and always wore his sword and boots. With them came 18 naval junior officers who often arrived in uniform but did not appear at all interested. But they were paying our bills.

And the last time she saw Usui-sama:

The following year we ran out of money again. O-Sensei departed for Fukuyama and we never saw him alive again. We all five stayed together after Usui's death. Hayashi took over the school and in May we moved to another temple. It was so sad!

Three Reiki Students in the Year 2001

In the first year of the twenty-first century, Chris Marsh, Andrew Bowling, and Taggart King began to present the world a very different picture of Reiki than we had previously received through Chujiro Hayashi and Hawayo Takata. This new picture emerged via direct contact between Chris Marsh and living students of Mikao Usui in Japan.

Chris Marsh is an English Reiki teacher and martial arts expert. He has been making trips to Japan for several decades, to further his study of martial arts. He speaks and reads Japanese and practices Tendai Buddhism. In the year 2000 he began to learn, through his martial arts teacher in Japan, that Mikao Usui, renowned for his Reiki healing system, had also been greatly revered as a martial artist.

At home in England, Chris contacted a fellow Reiki teacher, Andrew Bowling, to share this new discovery. The two became immediate friends and continued to receive information from Chris's teacher in Japan. In June of 2000, Chris made a trip to Japan for martial arts training. After the training was finished, he was introduced to a number of Reiki people, all of whom had been connected with Mikao Usui, and he was shown artifacts relating to Usui. Then he was introduced to a Buddhist nun, 106 years old. She was called Suzuki-san, and Usui himself had taught her his method. She began to teach Chris. She told him she was not happy with the way Reiki had come to be perceived and practiced in the world, and she wanted Usui's original teachings to be known again.

Chris returned to England and continued to receive information from Suzuki-san. A year later he went back to Japan, where he was met with an even greater surprise: This time he was introduced to eleven more of Usui's students, ranging in age from 96 to 111. Since then, he has continued to learn from them and has shared their teachings with Andrew Bowling and a third English Reiki teacher, Taggart King (no relation to Dave King), who has generously provided much of the information from Usui's living students presented in this book.

The Usui Gakkai

In 1926, after the passing of Mikao Usui, three of his final students were most likely involved in founding the URR Gakkai in Tokyo. There is no such official record; in fact, current members of the Gakkai maintain that Usui himself started the Gakkai in 1922. However, living students of Usui who are not members of the Gakkai say it was begun by a group of naval officers after Usui's passing, as a way of memorializing him.

The main impetus behind the creation of the Usui Gakkai was apparently Rear Admiral Jusaburo Ushida. Born the same year as Usui (1865), he was considerably older than the other officers—and some people credit Ushida alone with starting the Gakkai. Others say that two of his naval comrades, Kan'ichi Taketomi and Dr. Chujiro Hayashi, were also involved. That seems, to me, most likely.

On the stone at Usui's grave, Ushida is named as the calligrapher of the history presented there. He's also recorded as the second President of the Usui Gakkai (the first President allegedly being Usui). The third President was Ushida's fellow naval officer Kan'ichi Taketomi . . . and we can only wonder if their comrade Dr. Chujiro Hayashi would have been the next President had he not left the Gakkai in its early days, unhappy with changes that were being made in the teaching of Usui's method.

While it's easy to understand the creation of a memorial society as a way of honoring a departed Sensei, it's quite remarkable to me that people would create an official story of that person having been the founder and President of the Society, were it not true! And yet, it clearly seems that is what happened. There are, of course, many differences between Eastern and Western ways of thinking, and this appears to be an example of one. I was told that the naval officers felt there was greater honor to Usui if history recorded him as the founder and first President of the Society. Nonetheless, it seems the time has come to revise that history.

Even if Usui had started the Gakkai himself, it almost inevitably would have transformed after his passing. Certainly, what we know of the Gakkai today seems out of step with what we know of Usui. While everyone's version of Usui paints him as a very large presence (physically as well as spiritually), and as one who was quite open and giving and reaching out to others, the Gakkai that bears his name has a reputation for secrecy and exclusivity. It's a very small and closed organization. No one on the outside really knows what goes on inside; and no one gets inside unless invited by someone who is already a member. Not exactly the kind of organization we would associate with a man who went to great lengths to ensure that his gift to humanity was available to all.

It has been reported that membership in the Usui Gakkai is quite beneficial to one's visibility and position in the business and social strata of Tokyo—which, again, seems just the opposite of Usui's down-to-earth inclusiveness. And this may have been the nature of the Gakkai since its very beginning. We know that Dr. Hayashi left the Gakkai early on because he didn't like the changes that were being made to Usui's teachings; and one of his students, a Mr. Tatsumi, who also left the Gakkai after a short time, described it as an "officers' club."

To my knowledge, no one in the Reiki world outside Japan even learned of the Gakkai's existence until the 1990s. At this writing, only one member of the Gakkai—Hiroshi Doi—has come out of Japan and shared his knowledge of Japanese Reiki with the rest of us.

The Usui Gakkai has operated more or less continuously in Japan since its beginning. Immediately after World War II, during American occupation of Japan, the Gakkai was prohibited from meeting openly—it was apparently still a military "officers' club," which the Americans considered a security risk—but this is not to say the meetings did not continue secretly.

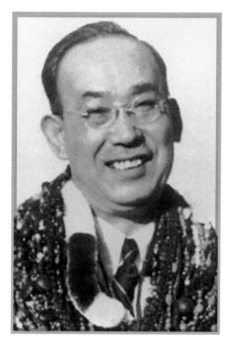

Dr. Chujiro Hayashi
Image courtesy Ann Fredholm
(http://users.pandora.be/annreiki/)

Dr. Chujiro Hayashi

Dr. Chujiro Hayashi was forty-seven years old, a retired Captain in the Japanese Navy, when he started training with Mikao Usui in May 1925. He and fellow naval officers Ushida and Taketomi are said to have been Usui's final students. It's believed that Usui met them while giving healings at a naval base, and that Hayashi convinced him to accept the three officers as his students. They were not characteristic of his other students, and some of Usui's friends are even said to have been upset that he would teach his spiritual method to military men. Hayashi was a medical doctor, and it seems the navy men were looking for something that could be used as a kind of First Aid for wounded warriors.

As it turned out, the now-famous Reiki symbols were introduced, in the final year of Usui's life, for the benefit of these navy officers. Usually students learned to incorporate certain elements of the teaching by practicing either Buddhist meditations or Shinto *kotodama* (sacred sounds).[20] But these navy men were taught symbols instead—maybe due to their religious beliefs,[21] or maybe as a way of expediting their learning process.

Dr. Hayashi had only about nine months of training from Usui—the final months of Usui's life. The students who have taught Chris Marsh say that was not enough time for Hayashi to learn the whole system as they learned it.[22] They say, for instance, that Hayashi learned the Reiju procedure after the formation of the URR Gakkai, probably from Toshihiro Eguchi. Dr. Hayashi was apparently involved in the beginning of the Gakkai but left it early on, by 1931 at the latest.

Following Usui's passing, Hayashi took charge of Usui's dojo and moved it to a different area of Tokyo (Shinano Machi). With the help of Taketomi and Ushida, he taught original Usui methods there and operated a hospice. In 1931 he changed the name to Hayashi Reiki Kenkyu-kai (Hayashi Reiki Research Center) and began teaching in his own way (which caused his student Tatsumi and others to separate from him).

In 1935 Hawayo Takata came to his clinic to be healed, then became his student. She returned home to Hawai'i, and Dr. Hayashi certified her in 1938, in Honolulu, as a "Master of Dr. Usui's Reiki system of healing." Their relationship and their personal philosophies would define Reiki outside Japan for the remainder of the twentieth century.

At his home on May 10, 1940, in front of his family and a group of his Reiki students (including Takata, who had made an urgent trip from Hawai'i at his request), Dr. Hayashi took his own life by *seppuku* (ritual slitting of the *hara*)—saying he was a peaceful man and could not go to war (he knew that he would be ordered back to military service in World War II).

Reiki Goes West: Hawayo Takata

Reiki didn't begin to reach the world outside Japan until just before World War II. At that time it spread to Hawai'i in the person of Hawayo

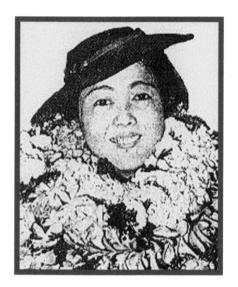

Hawayo Takata
Image courtesy http://johreiki.net/

Takata, an American woman of Japanese ancestry who had been healed of serious illness at Dr. Hayashi's Reiki clinic in Tokyo.

Ms. Takata was an American citizen by birth. She was named in honor of Hawai'i. She was born on the island of Kaua'i, on Christmas Eve, 1900. Her family name was Kawamuru; she married Saichi Takata in 1917. They had two daughters. In 1930 Saichi became very ill, went to Japan for treatment, and died there.

Five years later Hawayo went to Japan, quite ill herself. Her intent was to have surgery; then she received an intuition that it was not necessary and was directed to Dr. Hayashi's Reiki clinic for treatment. After recovering her health, she became a student of Reiki and was later certified a teacher. Naturally, what she learned was Hayashi's version of Reiki—and she may not have known the story of the Usui Gakkai, or even that it existed.

In 1940 she was present at her teacher's home in Japan to witness his ritual suicide—Hayashi's way of avoiding military service in World War II. By then, Takata had begun teaching the lower levels of Reiki, but she did not initiate any teachers until much later, 1976. In the late '70s, she traveled and taught[23] throughout the U.S., producing twenty-two Reiki teachers. It was through them and their students that Reiki began to spread around the globe.

The familiar "history" of Reiki—that it was the healing method of Jesus, rediscovered by Usui in the mid-1800s; that Usui himself was a Christian; that the Reiki symbols were divinely revealed to him in great, glowing balls of light, etc.—was the creation of Takata herself or with help from Dr. Hayashi. Understandably, this tale may have been necessary at the time of its invention: Imagine trying to interest Americans—especially in Hawai'i—in anything from Japan, in the days and years following the attack on Pearl Harbor, and the subsequent War! It's a miracle to me that Ms. Takata was able to get Reiki accepted then, with any connection to Japan whatsoever.

Apparently she did believe that Hayashi alone had been chosen to represent Reiki after Usui's passing. In like manner, she took that responsibility herself after Hayashi's passing. Indeed, in the 1970s she advertised herself as the "only Reiki Master in the world." At some point she began to be referred to as the "Grand Master of Reiki"—and, nearing the end of her life, started to look for her own successor. She chose her granddaughter Phyllis Furumoto,[24] but Phyllis was not interested. Takata persisted, until Phyllis eventually accepted the role of successor and was certified a Reiki Master by her grandmother.

Hawayo Takata left this world in December 1980, almost exactly eighty years after she entered it. Even after her departure, she continued to be—at least through the end of the twentieth century—the single greatest, defining influence on the practice of Reiki in the world at large.

In 1983, Phyllis Furumoto and other students in Takata's lineage created The Reiki Alliance, a global organization to spread their version of Reiki.

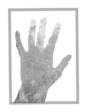

Chapter 2

Precepts, Concepts, Empowerment

The Reiki Precepts or Concepts

One of the very few items—and the only piece of writing—known today to be directly from the hand of Mikao Usui is a small scroll containing a single block of calligraphy. The few lines of advice presented there have long been called the Reiki Precepts. However, Melissa Riggall was told by Tenon-in that they are more accurately called "concepts" or "affirmations" (from the Japanese word *gainen*) than "precepts"—so I will call them Concepts here.

The Reiki Concepts are the very basis—and I believe the most important part—of Usui's "method to achieve personal perfection." Their absolute simplicity and brevity may give a deceptive impression of their power. When they were given to me at the first level of training, I paid them little attention; my only interest was in the ability to transmit healing energy. At the second level they were presented again, and again I discounted their importance. It was only after receiving third-level empowerments (almost eight years later) that I felt drawn to the Concepts and began to appreciate their greatness. Now, as I write this, almost nine years later yet, I realize even more how absolutely crucial it is to incorporate these Concepts into our being.

As with much of the Reiki history, there are differing viewpoints on the origin of the Concepts, and even their meanings. Reiki lore from the time of Takata has been that Usui took them from the writings of the Meiji Emperor, whom he greatly admired. But now, the picture emerging through the Japanese students is that Usui was not such an admirer of the Emperor. Mr. Doi has speculated that the Concepts may have come from the book *Kenzen no Genri* ("Fundamentals of Wellness") by Dr. Suzuki Bizan, published in 1914. But Chris Marsh's information is that the Usui Concepts were inspired by those of a ninth-century Tendai branch of Shugendo ("Way of Cultivating Spiritual Powers").

Where Usui got them is not so important. Nor are the Concepts necessarily unique; many spiritual teachers of Usui's time taught similar principles. The important thing is the wisdom contained in these Concepts, and their power for transforming our lives when we truly embody them.

Various translations of the Usui Concepts have appeared over the years, in a multitude of Reiki books. One translation (in addition to the one presented below) can be seen in Chapter 5 of this book (in the section titled "The Usui Memorial").

Tenon-in told Melissa Riggall that the Concepts were written by Usui on a day in 1921, on a sheet of paper now displayed in a private shrine, the location of which is kept secret. (Both Chris Marsh and Dave King have been taken there; Dave says he was transported blindfolded, to preserve the secrecy.)

Over the years, translations of this document have gotten shorter and shorter. I like it that way! I figure the shorter it is, the less embellishment, the more true to the original intent. For that reason, I very much like the Dave King translation below:[1]

> The Secret Method of Inviting Blessings
> The Spiritual Medicine of Many Illnesses
>
> Today only
> Anger not
> Worry not
> Do your work with appreciation
> Be kind to people
>
> In your life, perform *gassho*[2] as your mind recalls
> (these Concepts)
> The Usui system for connecting with your ancestral self
> through the body-mind

[*This last line* ("Shin shin kaizen Usui Reiki Ryoho") *is the only place Mikao Usui is known to have used the phrase* Usui Reiki Ryoho. *And what he meant by it, says Dave, is* Usui system for connecting with your ancestral self. *Taggart King has a similar viewpoint on the purpose of Reiju (literally, "giving Spirit"): that the intent is to bring about the state of being that was present before birth, "when we were Divine essence in complete connection to the universe."*]

Dave King makes a point of saying that Reiki is not so much an *energy* as it is a *presence*—the presence of our ancestral self. In any case, whichever word we use, the whole Reiki system (the Concepts, and Reiju, and everything else) is designed to awaken us to our real Self, the One we have always been and always will be; and to our unity with Perfect Universal Spirit.

Let's explore what these Concepts mean:

Today only: This means, very simply, Live in the present! Be Here Now! Embody these Concepts at every moment!

Anger not: This is self-evident—but I prefer to state it without using the word *anger* (because even when we say *anger not,* the subconscious mind focuses on *anger*). I prefer to use the words *I AM PEACE.*

Worry not: Again, self-evident; and again, I prefer to re-state it. Worry is a kind of fear, a lack of faith in the providence of Life itself. So, I like the words *I AM FAITH.*

Do your work with appreciation: For one thing, it helps when we reach the point of understanding that any work we do is work done on the Self. Beyond that, as Dave explains, this Concept is about learning the Taoist principle of Not-doing, or Doing-without-doing; that is, learning to be guided by Universal Spirit more than by the personal, rational mind. There is also an element here of interacting with Nature, interacting with Life, in a grateful way. Maybe this can all be said as *I DO WITHOUT DOING, AND GRATEFULLY.*

Be kind to people: I like Dave's equating of kindness here with "empathy and awareness." Also, he makes the point that it's important to show as much kindness to ourselves as to others. We can say then, very simply, *I AM KIND.*

In your life, perform gassho as your mind recalls (these Concepts): This has previously been translated, almost always, as the idea that one should sit, with hands in gassho, morning and evening, chanting (and internalizing) the Concepts. The point is to make these Concepts truly a part of ourselves, to embody them. This is confirmed by a final bit of translation done by Melissa Riggall. She translated this line as meaning to embody these Concepts not just morning *and* night, but *from* morning *to* night—in other words, *constantly, all the time.*

Clearly, the idea is to incorporate the Reiki Concepts in ourselves totally. I feel this equates with the advice in the Christian Bible to "pray without ceasing" (1 Thessalonians 5:17 KJV). And with the advice of yogis/yoginis, Zen Masters, and others—to make every moment of life a meditation. It's about changing our whole being, our energetic vibration, to one that resonates with the greater Universe!

Reiki empowerments, at each level, are only starting points, initiations. They connect us to as much universal energy as we are able to handle at the time, and we determine our own course of evolution (or devolution) from there. We can increase our capacity by transmitting Reiki to ourselves and others (or we can say it this way: by being in a state of Reiki), by doing meditations and energy exercises, and by receiving repeated empowerments. The most important thing, though, is what kind of energy we generate ourselves, all the time. This is where the Concepts prove to be so important.

Everything we experience in life is drawn to us by the kind of energy vibration we're sending out. Thoughts and feelings and beliefs involving fear, worry, anger, criticism, ingratitude, etc., generate low-frequency vibrations, which give birth to unpleasant experiences (disease, injury, depression, difficulties of all sorts). In the same way, vibrations of tolerance and love, gratitude, joy, peace, and well-being bring us happy and prosperous lives.

Reiki is a high-frequency vibration, which accounts for its ability to bring healing and spiritual awakening. Indeed, as Mr. Doi says, "Reiki is wave of love!" But many times we unconsciously counter its benefits by spending our time in worry or fear or sadness or anger. The Reiki Concepts are constant reminders to free ourselves of those lower vibrations and stay on the wavelengths of faith, peace, gratitude, and kindness. *The Reiki Concepts make Reiki a way of life, not just a transmission of healing energy to be turned on and off.* Through living the Concepts, we also come to realize that all disease and healing are simply landmarks on our path of spiritual awakening.

Each of us can find a way of incorporating these Concepts every day into our fundamental state of being. I cannot overemphasize the power this has in transforming our lives.[3]

Reiki Empowerment

One definitive aspect of Usui Reiki is the energetic "empowerment" of the student by the teacher. The outward aspect of this procedure customarily includes hand movements: the teacher's hands placed in a sequence of locations in the student's aura. The purpose, as with everything in Reiki, is to bring about the unification of the personal *ki* and the Universal *Rei.*

Exploring the history of empowerment procedures in Reiki, we find ourselves in yet another mystery. Dave King and Chris Marsh, both of whom have been taught by people who were taught by Usui himself, have encountered such *different* teachings! It's not surprising that Usui would have varied his teachings to fit individual students, or that his own method and understanding would have changed with time—surely those are safe to assume. But the mystery engulfs even something as basic as whether Usui himself used and/or taught any sort of energetic empowerment procedure.

According to Dave King, Usui did *not.* In laying out the historical sequence of empowerment procedures,[4] Dave says the following:

- Usui himself used *no* energetic empowerment procedure, only a ceremonial "rite of passage" at each level of the Usui-do system.
- Usui's friend Eguchi used this same ceremony (known as Trans-

formation) when teaching the system called Usui Teáte (which he was allowed to teach in Usui's dojo).

- Eguchi, when teaching his *own* system—which was called Eguchi Te-no-hira Ryoji (Eguchi Palm-of-the-hand Healing), and which he also taught in Usui's dojo—used an energetic empowerment procedure called *denju* ("instruction" or "initiation").

- Usui's students Ushida and Taketomi (the navy Admirals) were instrumental in deriving (from Usui Teáte) the method called Usui Reiki Ryoho, in which they used an energetic empowerment procedure called *Reiju* ("blessing" or "giving Spirit," which Dave believes was derived from Eguchi's *denju* procedure).

- Dr. Hayashi, around 1931, modified Usui's Transformation ceremony—and later replaced it with an energetic empowerment procedure called *Jikiden* ("initiation" or "direct transmission of skill").

- And, finally, that Hawayo Takata modified the Jikiden procedure to create what has come to be called Attunement.

We know, from Dave King and Mr. Doi and others, that Reiju has been used in the Usui Gakkai since its inception. But did Usui himself use Reiju? Dave says no. Chris Marsh's teachers say they received an energetic "blessing" or Reiju from Usui—but that he gave it without a formal procedure, just by intent. And that they were taught to give it using a formal Reiju procedure from Tendai Buddhism.

Could it be that the Reiju procedure, like Reiki symbols and kotodama and hand positions, was intended as "training wheels"—to be used as long as needed, and then put aside? Many of us have discovered for ourselves that there comes a time when Reiki "empowerment" can be given by mere intent, with no procedure at all. And now we learn that was indeed Usui's way of doing it.

More and more, I see that everything in Reiki is about one very simple aim: the bringing together (unification) of Universal Spirit *(Rei)* and a particular individual expression of that Spirit in the form of personal *ki.* Or we could say the unification of Yang and yin, Universal Wave and individual particle. In a word, Self-realization.

From what we know of Mikao Usui now, it seems that he must have reached such proficiency in this unification that his very presence would have shifted the energetic reality of others in a large and beneficial way. And that is exactly the intent with any kind of Reiki "empowerment"— to achieve the unification of *Rei* and *ki* in ourselves, and to pass that state of being to someone else.

The Chris Marsh information, via Taggart King,[5] is that Reiju was routinely given to people who came to Usui for healing. Some of those people then became students, and Reiju—received frequently—was an important contributor to their progress.

In the Usui Gakkai, Reiju is given to students at every meeting (according to Mr. Doi). The exact procedure may be slightly different than the one learned by Chris Marsh's teachers. Mr. Doi himself teaches yet another form of Reiju, in his Gendai (Modern) Reiki system. Gendai Reiju is only slightly different in procedure than what I learned as the Usui version. But to me there is a great difference in feeling between the two; and recipients have reported feeling a difference also.

One difference worth mentioning between Reiju and Attunement: Reiju is customarily given often and regularly (for example, weekly), while Attunement is typically given only once at each level of training. Attunement is intended to "open the Reiki connection" permanently; therefore, it is supposed, once is enough.

This distinction tells us something about the difference between Eastern and Western views of Reiki overall. The Eastern view sees Reiki as a lifelong process of growth; the Western view prefers to see it more as a one-time, permanent acquisition.

To me, the giving and receiving of frequent "empowerments" makes more sense. I cannot say that a Reiki Attunement is *not* a permanent opening of the Reiki connection, but I find such a statement not very meaningful. And it brings to mind an old joke, from way back in my childhood: A father announces to his son, "My boy, a job well done need never be done again!"—and the son says, "You mean ... like mowing the lawn?"

Yes, I feel it does help to mow the lawn often—whether physical or spiritual. And the words of my long-ago Latin teacher also come back to me: *"Repetitio iuvat!"* ("Repetition helps!")

In first-level Reiki *(Shoden),* Hawayo Takata used four Attunements. I wondered for a long time, Why four? Eventually I received an intuitive answer, later confirmed by another teacher. It seems that each of the four Attunements relates to a different "body" or aspect of our being—the physical, the mental, the emotional, and the spiritual— and that each corresponds with one of the four inner aspects of Reiki. These aspects are presented at second level *(Okuden)* and third level *(Shinpiden).*

Since Takata, many Reiki teachers have created their own forms of Attunement. Many use only a single Attunement where Takata used four. And, as mentioned above, there comes a time when we realize that Reiki empowerment can be given with no procedure at all, just by intent. It can also be given remotely, through time and space, as can Reiki "treatment." (Some people disagree with this, but I have many students in many countries, empowered at great distances, who attest to its effectiveness.)

What Is True Healing?

Mikao Usui taught that Reiki is both a spiritual healing technique and an energy healing technique, and he made a distinction between the two. Spiritual healing works at the fundamental level and affects Universal consciousness, while energy healing centers on removing symptoms from the individual mind and body.

Symptoms of illness or imbalance are important messages along our path of spiritual awakening. Energy healing alone can remove the symptoms, but true healing occurs only with a change of consciousness at the spirit level. Without such a change, we eventually replay the same symptoms or create different ones with the same message. Reiki not only balances our personal energies, it harmonizes our vibration with that of the greater Universe, which brings fundamental changes of consciousness and true healing.

Also, what appear to be symptoms of illness may in truth be the healing process itself. True healing requires that toxins in the body be either transmuted or released; if not transmuted into something useful, then they must be purged from the body. This occurs whether the toxins are physical, mental, emotional, or spiritual—so we may experience their departure as a change of consciousness, an emotional release (feelings of anger, sadness, anxiety, for example), or as physical discharges.

In using Reiki, we see the best results when we keep in mind that we are not the ones doing the healing, we are merely a focal point for the universal energy. We simply welcome the energy and let it flow through us. We make no effort to control the results. Our intent is to put aside our personal desires, to get ourselves out of the way, to let the Reiki flow as cleanly as possible through us.

The Importance of Intent and the Danger of Ego

The most important thing in life (besides breathing!) is intent. Even if there are mistakes and deficiencies in our technique, a good intent will usually accomplish the desired result. Intent is primary, and comes from the heart; technique is secondary, and comes from the head and hands.

What is our intent when using Reiki? Is it to remove symptoms, or to achieve any sort of predetermined outcome? Or is it simply to open the connection to Source, to increase the flow of Source energy, trusting the best outcome to follow naturally? My experience has shown that as soon as I think I'm doing something, what I'm really doing is giving my ego a pat on the head, and the best results occur when I'm not-doing.

My not-doing may include the use of some technique—for instance, in a Reiki session, or in giving Reiju—but I see the technique as only a doorway for the Source energy (which is responsible for any doing that occurs). Sometimes no technique is involved at all—and, remarkably, those are almost always the times when the greatest things happen!

I do Reiju with people all over the world, every day. I ask them to pick the day and time they prefer to receive the Reiju, and I write their information (name, location, date, and time) on a piece of paper. Then, sometimes, it happens that I get so busy with other things, the time for someone's Reiju comes and goes without my remembering to do the Reiju. Sometimes I find the written note after the time has passed, and I do the Reiju then (still intending that it be perceived by the other person at their chosen time). But, other times, what reminds me of the Reiju is an email in my Inbox, telling me how wonderful/powerful/spectacular the Reiju was!

I feel sure these descriptions are not the results of wild imaginings; they're too varied and genuine-sounding for that, and they often include tangible, quantifiable evidence. So, how can it be that someone "receives" a Reiju that I forgot to "send"?

The only answer I can see is that the Reiju was carried out through the combination of my initial intent, written on the paper, and the intent of the recipient—that it was a "done deal" from the moment we agreed on the day and time of it! And, for my part, many instances have shown me that putting my intent in writing is not even necessary; the intent can be conveyed instantly and wordlessly.

The danger of ego is that it constricts the flow of Reiki (our "highest ki"), and it constricts the flow of Source energy. The ego is much too narrow a conduit for these energies!

Sometimes we are given intuitive knowledge of a person's condition, or of a specific technique or action or piece of advice that will help them; but it's important that we learn to distinguish between intuition and ego. If thinking is involved, we're probably dealing with ego. Intuition, at least in my experience, is thoughtless, wordless, and lightning-fast: a silent, sudden knowing. Any concepts of something being "wrong," something needing to be "fixed," are definitely coming from the ego. Instead of trying to "fix" anything, we can merely open the flow of Source energy, which will accelerate the fulfillment of the original intent embodied in the person. Another way to say it is: We're connecting the person with his or her real Self—which does not require our ego to be thinking or doing anything.

Here's a real-life example of ego getting in the way (and in a more subtle way than what we often think of as ego):

Once, when I was teaching someone how to give Reiju, I was the recipient, and I was describing the procedure, step-by-step, as the giver

was going through the motions. This was strictly a "practice run": Th
giver didn't need to know anything in advance, wasn't trying to remember anything, was just doing what I told her to do. At every position
of her hands, I was feeling a great amount of energy flowing, and so
was she.

After the "practice run" we did a Reiju "for real": This time she
had to remember all the steps; this time she was thinking about doing
everything right, and about impressing the teacher; and this time ...
both of us felt almost no energy flowing at all!

Another way the ego sometimes intrudes is by camouflaging itself
as love and compassion. I don't mean that we should not have love
and compassion—only that, sometimes, people give their love and
compassion instead of Reiki. Some people are so compassionate, they
don't know how to keep from giving away their personal energy! A
sure sign of this happening is that the person feels tired or "drained"
after giving a healing session, instead of feeling more energized than
before the session.

It may be hard to see this as a form of ego, but it is—it's a lack of
trust in the Reiki and in the Source energy of the recipient; a feeling
that the "giver" must personally accomplish the healing (and also, possibly, the desire to take credit for it).

This brings up another point, which I believe is extremely important. It goes back to intent: If our intent is only to give energy—even
Reiki—from an outside source, then the recipient tends to become
dependent on continued applications of this energy. But if our intent
is to use the Reiki to open the flow of the recipient's own Source energy,
from within ... hmmm ... Who knows what that might accomplish?

Different Approaches to Reiki

In the past there has been a fundamental difference between Japan and the rest of the world in the perception of Usui Reiki and the attitude toward it. In Japan, Reiki has been practiced as a spiritual path; the physical healing effects were seen, accurately, as secondary. Reiki was a lifetime practice requiring devotion and a sense of reverence, and the goal was to attain "personal perfection," not primarily to heal others. Usui himself did give healings, but he also empowered his patients so they could heal themselves.

The Western approach has viewed Reiki mainly as a way of healing the physical body, an alternative or an adjunct to pills or surgery or any other sort of treatment. Reiki came to the West through Hayashi and Takata: a medical doctor, whose focus was very much on the physical healing of others, and one of his patients who was healed. It's hard to imagine that, in those days, the Western mentality would have accepted any other manifestation of Reiki.

Another characteristic difference relates to Reiki training. As we're learning from Usui's living students, the training was ongoing, and it was usual for them to spend several months meditating on a single aspect. Only when it was clear that one element had been fully incorporated were they introduced to the next. It has been this way in the Usui Gakkai also, where students are sometimes held at one level for many years.

The Western approach has generally centered on sharply defined classes or workshops, presenting an entire level of training in a weekend or a single day. Naturally, this feature came to us via Dr. Hayashi also. His emphasis was not on spiritual development; he was training people to give a simple healing treatment. In the late 1920s, we know, he was giving Shoden and Okuden training together in five consecutive days (and only two hours or less per day).

In Western-style Reiki, this trend has persisted. Some teachers even give all three levels, claiming to make people Reiki Masters, in a single weekend. Personally, I believe a longer period of time is necessary to allow assimilation of each new level of energy, to undergo personal changes brought on by the new vibrations, and to learn by practicing with the Reiki itself. (Just as it's not effective to give a small potted plant a gallon of water at once—most of the water cannot be held and simply runs away, and sometimes the plant can even be drowned.)

There's also the element of money. When I think of Mikao Usui, I keep hearing the words, "available to everyone." I believe that was indeed his intention for his Reiki method. Hawayo Takata told an elaborate story about Usui declaring the necessity of receiving something in exchange for Reiki, a lesson he had supposedly learned after seven years of giving Reiki freely in the slums of Kyoto.[6] Much has been said about this "rule" of "energy exchange." I've often heard it described as "People don't value anything they don't have to pay for"—and its corollary is "The more they have to pay, the more they value something."

This was apparently the paradigm in which Hayashi was operating when, around 1928, he was charging the modern-day equivalent of approximately US$5,000 for his combination Shoden-Okuden class. And it was a paradigm embraced and propagated by Takata, who charged US$10,000 for Master attunement, and by The Reiki Alliance, which followed her.

I personally also believe in "energy exchange." But I believe it's as natural as breathing. It's the way the universe operates inevitably, it's not something we have to make happen. Whenever we breathe out, we have no choice but to breathe in immediately; and whatever kind of energy we send out into the universe is what comes back to us. It can be no other way.[7]

Mikao Usui wanted the Reiki connection made available to all, and evidence suggests that his services were offered freely or for minimal fees. (This was also the case with Usui's friend Eguchi, who sometimes taught his own healing method at Usui's dojo. According to Andrew Bowling, when Eguchi later joined the Usui Gakkai, money was at least part of the reason he did not remain a member for long. He complained of the high membership fees there, in addition to disliking the military atmosphere.)

It's ironic that Reiki, until recent years, had almost vanished from the land of its birth, even as it was burgeoning elsewhere. Usui's remaining students were dwindling in number, and apparently not much interested in spreading their knowledge. The Usui Gakkai continued teaching its own version of Reiki, but so secretively that its existence was (and still is) hardly known even in Tokyo. (Members refuse to tell outsiders even the location of the building!) Then, even more ironic, when Reiki was re-introduced in Japan in the 1990s, it was by foreigners teaching Western-style Reiki.

Now, as we enter the Aquarian Age, some of these long-isolated Reiki streams are beginning to flow together. And we're finding gold in them—especially in the teachings of those who were taught by Usui himself.

Degrees or Levels

From Hiroshi Doi we have descriptions of Shoden, Okuden, and Shinpiden levels in the Gakkai. We also know there is a final level, Shihan

(Teacher). In the West, many Reiki teachers also teach four levels, roughly equivalent with the Japanese levels:

1. Shoden (The Entrance): This gives a general awakening to the Reiki energy. The emphasis at this level is usually on self-treatment.

2. Okuden (The Deep Inside): The student is given conscious awareness of three particular aspects within Reiki; the capacity for transmitting Reiki is generally enhanced; and the emphasis in treatment may shift from self to others.

3. Shinpiden (The Mystery): This involves conscious awareness of a fourth aspect, which incorporates the other three and gives the student the ability to initiate others to transmit Reiki. It also greatly increases one's own Reiki capacity.

4. Shihan (Teacher): As the name says, this level is for those who want to teach.

In Western Reiki, this fourth level is a fairly recent addition. When I received the first two levels, in 1991 from a member of The Reiki Alliance, there were only three levels. The third was often called Reiki Master, and the word "master" meant "teacher." No one was initiated into that level unless they committed themselves to teaching Reiki. When I received my third-level initiation, in 1999 from an independent teacher, she followed the same system. But in recent years the title of Master seems to have no connection with teaching. It has come to mean anyone who is pursuing "personal perfection"—to use Mikao Usui's own description—through Reiki.

The term "Reiki Master" has sometimes caused confusion, with people taking it to mean that someone has "mastered" Reiki. What we learn, though, after practicing Reiki for some time, is that the only thing one can ever master is oneself. Reiki is one of countless ways of doing that—and we also discover that self-mastery is indeed an endless journey. People need to understand that "Reiki Master" means only that someone has been *initiated* into the third level of Reiki. Nowadays the term "Master Teacher" or "Master/Teacher" is often used for a person who teaches Reiki. And some of us prefer just the word "teacher," to avoid confusion.

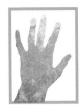

Chapter 3

Doing-Without-Doing

Giving Reiki

I believe the most important thing in Reiki, aside from living the Concepts, is the practice of Reiki self-treatment. I see Reiki as an "extension cord" to our Source, therefore to the truth of us, our genuine, original, and eternal Self (which is expressed only to a limited degree through the persona, the *mask* of any physical lifetime). I believe the primary effect of Reiki is to accelerate our discovery of the reality of ourselves. As with the Concepts, I cannot overemphasize the importance of Reiki self-treatment. I give myself Reiki for at least an hour every day (preferably before getting out of bed in the morning).[1]

Before I describe this treatment, let's look at the concept of *chakras*. It's a concept that may or may not have been utilized by Usui, having originated in India (though, considering the type and range of his knowledge, it's hard to imagine that he would not have encountered it). In Japan, a system of energy meridians was the basis of hands-on healing methods (as well as acupuncture) long before the arrival of Usui Reiki. In any case, the classic Indian chakra system works beautifully with Reiki and is infinitely simpler than the network of meridians.

Chakra is a Sanskrit word meaning "wheel." Chakras are wheels of subtle energy, usually unseen by most of us, that empower the workings of our human bodies. We contain hundreds of chakras (at least), including seven primary ones in the physical body itself.[2]

People who see chakras have described these seven in a line from the base of the spine to the crown of the head, as follows:

1. Root or Base Chakra: at the perineum, between the genitals and anus. Associated with the color Red, element Earth, planet Earth, and with family/tribal identity.

2. Sacral Chakra: slightly below the navel. Associated with the color Orange, element Water, the Moon, and with survival and reproduction, personal power, creativity, and one-to-one relationships.

3. Solar Plexus Chakra: above the navel, in the solar plexus. Associated with the color Yellow, element Fire, the Sun, and with self-esteem and personal identity.

4. Heart Chakra: in the center of the chest. Associated with the color Green (and sometimes Pink or Salmon), element Air, and with the overall health and balance of body and spirit.

5. Throat Chakra: at the base of the throat, just above the clavicle. Associated with the color Blue, element Akasha (or vibration, manifestation), and with choice, faith, and self-expression.

6. Brow Chakra: between and just above the eyebrows, and sometimes called the Third Eye. Associated with the color Indigo (or Violet), and with intuition, reason, and evaluation.

7. Crown Chakra: at the crown of the head. Associated with the color Violet (or White), and with the integration of our spirituality. This is considered to be the gateway between the energies of the material Universe and the purely spiritual energy of Divine Source.

The chakras provide and regulate the energy responsible for our living. And the chakras are activated by two fundamental energies, known as *yang* and *yin*.[3] These come to us from Heaven and Earth (respectively), and we may picture them empowering the seven major chakras in the following way: Heaven energy spiraling down, entering our body at the Crown Chakra; Earth energy spiraling up, entering our body at the Root Chakra (in addition to the countless whirlpools of yin-yang arising throughout our energy field).

People who see the chakras describe a funnel-shape of energy at the Crown, and an upside-down funnel-shape at the Root. Heaven energy descends through a channel on one side of the spine—entering at the Crown, engaging chakras Six through Two as it moves downward, then leaving through the Root. Earth energy ascends through a channel on the other side of the spine—entering at the Root, engaging chakras Two through Six as it moves upward, then leaving through the Crown.

Given the chakras' positions between these two oppositely flowing streams of energy, the spinning of the interior chakras is greatly enhanced. The streams of yin and yang make them spin, and energy is drawn into them from the back of the body and sent out the front—forming a pair of energy-funnels (one in back, one in front) at each of the chakras Two through Six.

Now we're ready for my favorite form of self-Reiki. . . .

You Are The Universe!

The procedure is to lie on my back and put hands on the head, down to the throat, then continue straight down the middle of the body. This treats the seven major chakras, of course, and through them the whole body.

One day as I was doing this, I had a realization about the relationship of the human body to the greater Universe—how the human body is indeed a microcosm of the macrocosmic Universe (which I had known intellectually before but had not really felt in a deep way). I experienced the feeling of a holographic Universe, and the fact that our tiny human bodies actually encompass All That Is. I felt this as the true essence of Reiki: the union of Universal Spirit *(Rei)* and personal energy *(ki)*. It's the realization that we encompass, and can affect, everything in the Universe; and that we can focus the wisdom and power of the whole Universe through our personal bodies.

As I held my hands on my head and then started moving them down the rest of the body, I began to see the human system—specifically the major chakras—as a reflection of our solar system:

Crown Chakra: the gateway to the energy of Heaven.

Brow Chakra: The stillness of One becomes the first stirrings of Two, the inseparable yin and yang, whose interaction creates everything in the dualistic Universe. (Time and space are the first two.)

Throat Chakra: Let there be Light—and ten thousand other things! The will, the voice, the Word—precipitating concrete manifestation from the swirls of chaos.

Heart Chakra: the element of Air (which empowers and governs the human heart and lungs). The energy of Breath. The Atmosphere of planet Earth.

Solar Plexus Chakra: the element of Fire (which empowers and governs the stomach, liver, gall bladder, spleen, and pancreas). The energy of Digestion, Alchemy, Transmutation. The Sun.

Sacral Chakra: the element of Water (which empowers and governs the intestines, kidneys, urinary bladder, reproductive organs).[4] The energy of Assimilation, Relationship, Two-becoming-One in sacred union (resulting in a new creation). The Moon.

Root Chakra: the element of Earth. The fundamental energy of physical existence. The rock and soil of planet Earth.

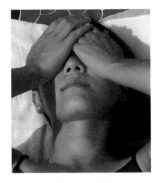

Having this awareness, we can consciously connect with these energies in their totality, as they make up the whole Universe. The human body is a hologram of All That Is, and as we give Reiki to ourselves we can direct it, via these elements, throughout all creation.

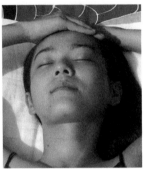

I start with palms over eyes, the fingers of each hand crossing over the Brow Chakra[5]....

Then move them one at a time to cover the crown....

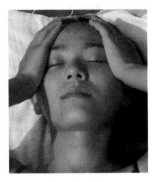

Then temples....

Then the front of the face (bottoms of palms at the jaw line, fingers covering eyes)....

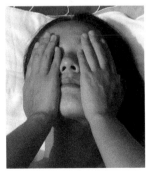

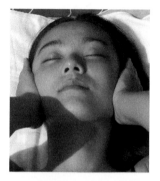

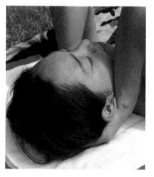

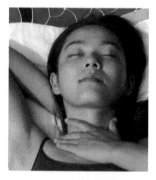

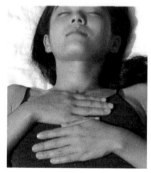

Then ears. . . .

Then back of head. . . .

Then move the right palm to the back of the throat chakra (fifth cervical vertebra), and the left palm to the front of the throat chakra (magnetism and manifestation). . . .

Then put the right hand on the front, immediately below the left hand . . . and move the left hand down, immediately below the right hand. The top edge (thumb) of the right hand is now at the top of the sternum, and the bottom edge (little finger) of the left hand is at the bottom of the sternum. This covers the heart chakra (element of Air) and the heart and thymus and lungs. . . .

Then move the right hand down, just below the left, and the left hand down below the right again. The top edge of the right hand is now at the bottom of the sternum, and the bottom edge of the left hand is at the navel. This covers the solar plexus chakra (element of Fire) and associated organs. . . .

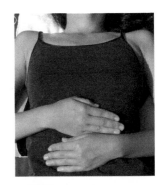

Then move the right and left hands down in the same way again, so the top edge of the right hand is at the navel and the bottom edge of the left hand is at the pubic bone. The sacral chakra (element of Water) and associated organs are covered here. . . .

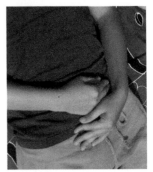

Then, with both hands, cover the root chakra (element of Earth), between genitals and anus. This can be done by bringing the knees up, heels against buttocks, and reaching both hands down in front, or by turning the body on its side (fetal position) and reaching one hand down in front and the other in back. . . .

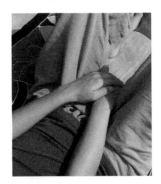

Then I leave one hand at the root chakra and move the other up to the crown chakra and let Reiki flow all the way between them, descending from Heaven . . . through Time and Space . . . into the world of Manifestation . . . through Air . . . through Fire . . . through Water . . . to Earth; and then feel the ascension, from Earth to Water to Fire to Air . . . to Magnetism, to Space-Time, to Source. (As you go through this whole sequence, you might also like to experiment with feeling Tree energy at the navel, between Fire and Water.)

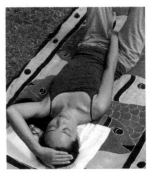

This method of self-Reiki can also be used to send Reiki simultaneously to individuals and to the whole world. With your hands in the first position (over eyes), visualize or feel yourself connecting with individual recipients—for the greatest healing, awakening, empowerment of each—to be received whenever each person is most receptive within the next twenty-four hours.

Then simply feel the Reiki as you move your hands through all the positions. You can put your attention on individual recipients at each position, or not—knowing that Reiki is flowing to fill each recipient you've connected with, as well as yourself, as well as the greater Universe. As you move through the positions, feel the Reiki flowing in sequence through every aspect: the connection with Heaven; the initial stirrings of yin and yang; the coalescing of elements; the energies of Air, Fire, Water, and Earth.[6]

I recommend spending at least half an hour on the head and half an hour on the body. (I find an hour of Reiki more restful and energizing than an hour of sleep.) Of course, if you must, you can do the whole treatment in as little time as necessary. Or you can do only part of it. If I have to choose between head and body, my tendency is usually to do only the head and throat.

Naturally, any time we have a pain or an injury, we can give Reiki by putting hands directly on the spot (or in the aura just above, if it's painful to touch). We can also give Reiki at various times during the day, whenever we're not busy, by putting one or both hands anywhere on the body. Reiki will be directed wherever it's most needed in the body.

I urge my students to give themselves as much Reiki as possible every day, especially in the weeks immediately following initiation into each level, in order to maximize the benefit of their new vibrations.

Treating Others

Reiki nowadays is generally given with the recipient lying down, which allows maximum relaxation, therefore maximum receptivity to the energy. We'll look at three different styles of reclining treatment, a couple of ways to give a sitting treatment, and a way of treating the seven major chakras by giving Reiki only to the hands.

General Procedure

First of all, prepare a clean, orderly, and peaceful space for the treatment. In addition to the physical setting, order and purify the subtle energy of the place. To prepare a nice energy, you can sit there and meditate on the Concepts for a few minutes, or just focus on your breathing, or ask that Reiki fill and overflow the space, creating an atmosphere of absolute safety and comfort, bringing the greatest awareness to you and the person you'll be treating.

I recommend having water available for drinking before, during, and after the treatment. When you prepare the space, you might like to pour a glass of water, wrap your hands around it, and sit there for a few minutes, letting Reiki fill the water, which the person can drink later.

Both giver and recipient should wear loose clothing made of natural fibers, so the body can relax and the skin can breathe. It's not necessary to remove clothing, as long as it fits loosely. Some people say it's important to remove jewelry, though I've not usually felt that myself. Let your intuition be your guide!

During treatment, your hands can rest lightly on the body or slightly above, in the aura. It's good to ask whether the recipient has a preference. In either case, the Reiki will be more concentrated if the fingers are held together. You may find yourself more sensitive to the energy flow when your hands are slightly above the body—though you may be able to relax more completely by resting the hands on the body. Also, most people find the physical contact comforting, a welcome addition to the Reiki. When contacting the body directly, you may find your sensitivity increased by cupping the hands just barely, to create a small airspace under the palm. When moving hands from one position to the next, do it slowly and smoothly, one at a time.

Whenever possible, wash your hands with soap and water before giving any kind of treatment, and always have a reverent attitude. The recipient and yourself are both extensions of Divine Source, about to engage in a loving and intimate exchange of energy.

Do your best always to position your body in the most balanced and relaxed way, to avoid holding yourself in place with muscle tension. This not only keeps you from becoming tired, it allows a better flow of Reiki.

After the treatment, offer the person water. Advise them that one effect of the Reiki will be to discharge toxins from the body; that they may notice this discharge in the form of emotions, or as physical symptoms such as coughing, sneezing, a runny nose, etc.—and that drinking plenty of water for the next few days will aid the process of cleansing.

The Tanden and the One Point

Just below the navel (where the umbilical cord connected us with our mother during our time in the womb) is a point commonly called the *tanden*. This point is seen as very important in martial arts—as the point where both mind and body are centered, considered by some to be the *source of ki* in the body. Viewing it as the center-point, and increasing our awareness of it, can be very helpful in flowing our life energy with least effort and greatest effect. This point is two or three finger-widths below the navel, and about the same distance inward.

I was taught that the word *tanden* is merely the Japanese equivalent of the Chinese *tan tien* or *dan tien*. However, I've recently been informed (thanks to Mike Fuchs, who teaches not only Reiki, but T'ai Chi and Chi-gung) that dan tien is really quite different than what we're talking about here as "the tanden."

Literally, both dan tien and tanden mean "red field"—though dan tien is commonly translated as "elixir field" (referring to a field in which the "elixir of life" is planted).

According to Mike, from the Chinese/Taoist viewpoint, the human body has not just one of these elixir fields, but three. There's a dan tien centered in the head, and one in the chest (the heart area), as well as the one in the abdomen. Some other sources describe the middle dan tien as being centered in the solar plexus instead of the heart area.

According to Mike, the dan tien in the abdomen extends from the solar plexus area clear down into the earth—so, these are not little fields. How, then, has the word "tanden" come to mean a single point instead of a larger field?

It may be just another example of the difference between Eastern and Western ways of thinking. But with a little more research, we see that *it appears to be simply a misnomer.*

All of the following are commonly used interchangeably: tanden, dan tien, tan tien … and then … *kikai tanden, seika tanden,* and *seika no itten.* Among these last three, *kikai tanden* means "ocean-of-ki red field," and *seika tanden* means "below-the-navel red field"—both clearly designating *fields,* not single points. Only the final description turns out to be the one we're looking for: *seika no itten,* meaning "the one point below the navel." *Wow!!*

This One Point is seen as the key to unification of body and mind. It's the center of gravity for the body, and it's where the focus of the mind should be held. Renowned Aikido Master Koichi Tohei teaches a beautiful way of experiencing this. First, he says, just relax the body; then feel that the whole universe is condensing into the body; then the body condenses into the One Point. The One Point should be the smallest point conceivable.

I feel this is not just an imaginary exercise, but the true awareness of what is really happening. All the elements of the greater Universe are being pulled into the gravitational *field* of the tanden—into the One Point—and then projected out from there to create the universe of the individual human body! Each of us really is a whole, expansive universe centered on One (super-gravitational) Point. My feeling is also that, as the elements are swirling from the external Universe into our One Point, they are simultaneously welling up from the Source-dimension *within* the One Point—welling up and being projected outward to create our personal universe.

When we keep the mind and body focused in the One Point, says Koichi Tohei, we are the strongest and also the calmest that we can be. In this calmness, we have the potential for limitless movement. Every movement should begin from this point, every outside influence be absorbed here.

By keeping mind and body centered in the One Point, we can truly relax both mind and body. When the weight of the whole body settles into the One Point, the body can relax, and the mind is then calm. In this state of relaxation and calmness, we are naturally and effortlessly balanced and aware, and our ki is extended.

Finding the One Point

Stand with feet shoulder-width apart, pelvis forward slightly, arms hanging loosely. Tuck the chin slightly inward. Holding the tip of your tongue on the roof of the mouth, just behind the teeth, inhale through the nose, down into the abdomen. Exhale through the mouth, letting the tongue drop down naturally. Take a few breaths, relax the body and, feeling as balanced as possible, focus your attention below the navel. Then move your body very slowly, either slightly upward (by rising straight up on the toes) or slightly downward (by bending the knees). This will help you feel a sensation in the One Point.

Sitting Treatment

Let's consider how to treat a seated recipient. Some people say that Usui generally preferred this position over lying down. They say he would give Reiki to the head for about a half hour, then on the body, only to spots where his hands were intuitively drawn. And that he recommended as a good general procedure treating the head, stomach, and intestines.

Another good treatment, whether sitting or lying, is a slight variation of the "You Are The Universe!" self-treatment. The recipient should sit as comfortably and balanced as possible. Before the session, you can ask if the person wants to talk about anything: what's happening in their life, why they've come for a Reiki session, etc. Allow them to say as little or as much as they desire; just listen carefully and respond according to your intuition. Do your best in all ways to put them at ease. It's not even necessary that they tell you anything, except to the extent that talking is a therapeutic release for them. In any case, the

Reiki will flow in whatever amount they are able to receive, working at all levels, physical, mental, emotional, and spiritual.

To start the treatment, I stand behind the seated recipient. I like to bring my hands together in gassho, and to stipulate, in my mind, that I be a clear conduit for the Reiki; that the greatest healing, awakening, empowerment be received. This can be in the form of a prayer, an affirmation, or whatever feels most natural to you—the idea is merely to be clear about your intent. You can also specify other qualities appropriate to the person's needs, such as Joy, Love, Prosperity, Generosity, Faith, Peace, Truth, Patience, Understanding, Wisdom, Purification, etc.

Then I like to smooth down the aura with my hands. Some people say this is absolutely crucial; others may not even do it. It does seem beneficial, if only as a gentle way of making the first tangible contact with the recipient.

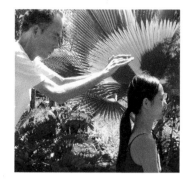

Standing behind them, I start with my hands above their crown and sweep gently down, almost to the ground. Moving to the right (in a counterclockwise circle around them), I repeat this until I'm back where I started, standing behind the person. (Going in the counterclockwise direction, I feel, has an "opening" effect.)

Sometimes I go around again, this time with fingers apart, "combing" down through the aura. Then one more time of smoothing. These techniques seem to remove knots of energy from the aura, something like smoothing tangles out of

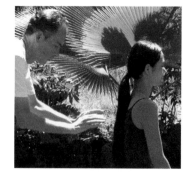

hair with a brush or a comb. Still, sometimes rough spots remain where I feel particular sensations in my hands: warmth or coolness, tingling, buzzing, dragging or sticking, even sharp or dull pains. I don't try to diagnose or analyze these, just notice them as places where the aura doesn't feel smooth. And I can feel again later, during the treatment, to see if things have changed.

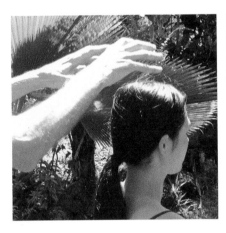 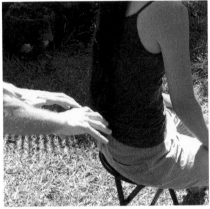

Now I move my hands through the following positions:

Right hand on back of head (occiput), left hand on forehead (middle finger at hairline), while standing at the person's left side.

Palms on temples (standing behind).

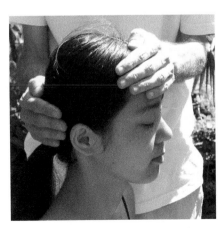 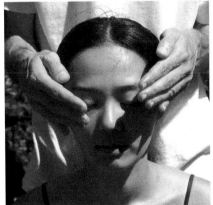

Palms on ears.

Palms on upper back of head (fingertips pointing upward; it helps to kneel for this one).

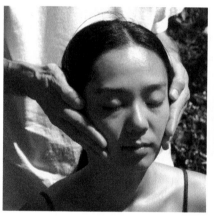 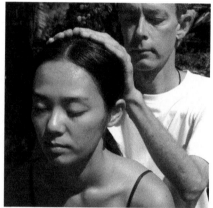

Palms on lower back of head and neck (still kneeling).

Palms on crown (standing behind again).

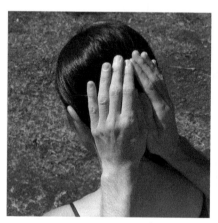 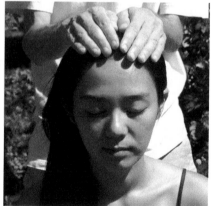

Right hand on back of throat chakra (fifth cervical vertebra), left hand on front (standing to left side).

Proceeding down from here, I can either do the front and back of each chakra, one by one—or in stair-steps, as follows:

With right hand still on back of throat chakra, move left hand to (or in front of) heart chakra.

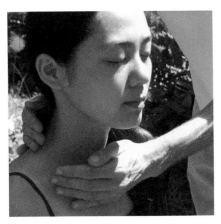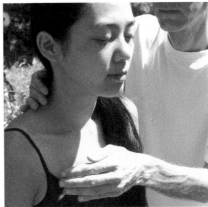

Move right hand to back of heart chakra, then left hand to front of solar plexus.

Move right hand to back of solar plexus, then left hand to front of sacral chakra.

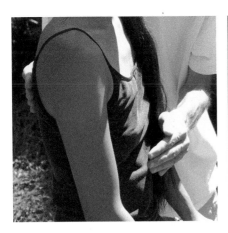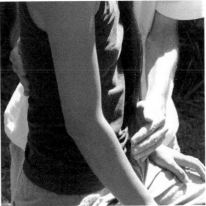

Move right hand to back of sacral chakra. Then move around to the front, putting a hand on each knee. (This can be done smoothly by bringing the left hand from sacral chakra to left knee, then replacing it with the right hand, moving the left one to the right knee.)

Move hands to ankles (thumb on one side of ankle, fingers on the other).

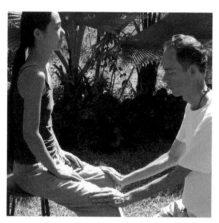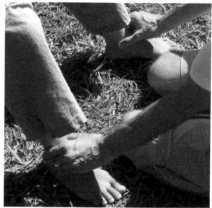

Hands on tops of feet (I like to visualize energy, like tree roots, going down through the feet, deep into the Earth, grounding the person).

Now I can move quickly from the feet, to a knee, to a shoulder, to standing behind the person, one hand on each shoulder, sending more

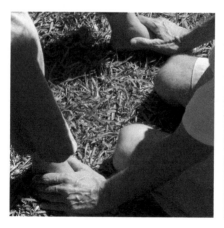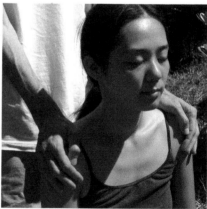

ADVENTURES OF DAVE AND MELISSA

Dave King and Melissa Riggall were Taoist Chi-gung students visiting Morocco in 1971 when they met Yuji Onuki, a student of Toshitoro (a.k.a. Toshihiro) Eguchi. Eguchi himself had been a close friend and student of Mikao Usui in Japan in the 1920s. In 1971, Dave knew nothing of Reiki or Usui's connection with it (his introduction to Reiki would come twenty-one years later in Canada). From Eguchi's student in Morocco, however, he and Melissa began to learn "a simple but powerful system that used *qi* (chi) in a mindful yet unconditional manner and without the endless work needed" in regular Chi-gung.[7]

Following his 1992 initiation into Reiki, Dave and Melissa made several trips to Japan. They spent a good deal of time learning from a student of Dr. Hayashi, a Mr. Tatsumi. Between 1927 and 1931, Tatsumi said, he learned from Hayashi what Hayashi had learned from Usui. He allowed Dave and Melissa to copy his notes, including the Reiki symbols in Hayashi's own handwriting.

For years, in Toronto, Dave and Melissa taught the traditional Japanese techniques they had learned (under the name of Usui-do) and continued making trips to Japan. Melissa in particular met and spent time with many students of Hayashi, Eguchi, and Usui (twenty-nine in all). Eventually she went to live at a Taoist retreat center in China. She passed away there in 2003, having been given the name Shen-Lissa three years earlier. In 2004, Dave moved to China, closing the dojo in Toronto.

grounding energy down through the shoulders, through the whole body, and into the Earth.

Finally, I sweep down the aura again, this time going clockwise for a "closing" effect. If I still feel rough spots, I can work intuitively to smooth them out as I go. Then I go around one final time, this time sweeping energy upward for an awakening, revitalizing effect. This finishes the treatment, though it's good for the person to remain seated a few minutes, "tuning in" to any revelations or intuitions received, and coming gently back to normal consciousness.

Reclining Treatment

Seven Positions

In the late 1990s, Dave King taught the following hand positions as a "Traditional Japanese Reiki" treatment. They are based on acupuncture meridians, primarily the gall bladder meridian. He says, "These positions are part of a standard healing pattern in use long before Usui's time"; and that Usui was using them in a healing system he created "around 1900." This was not Usui-do, which Dave says was taught by Usui from 1922 to 1925 and did not involve the healing of others.

Some of these hand positions use the fingertips to direct energy at certain meridian points on the body; these are points where energy naturally enters or leaves the meridian system.

Position 1: Eyes

Curl the fingertips and place them gently on the fleshy tissue just below each eye. The fingertips should be pointing directly downward (this requires short fingernails, to avoid causing discomfort in the recipient). Your palms can rest gently on the forehead. The entry points of the bladder, stomach, and gall bladder meridians are located around the eyes. These meridians terminate in the feet.

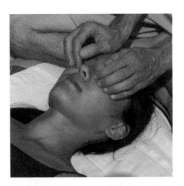

Position 2: Temples

Slowly lift one hand and place the tip of the thumb gently at the outside corner of the corresponding eye, where the eyebrow line would pass through if extended in its natural curve. Slowly move your other hand into position on the other side of the head. This position covers parts of the gall bladder and triple heater meridians.

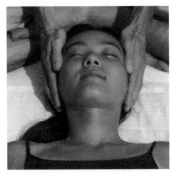

Position 3: Occiput

Apply a gentle suggestion of pressure to the left side of the head, and ask the recipient to roll the head to the side. This allows you to place your left hand on the back of the head (fingertips down near the neck area). Then gently roll the head back to the center position (using the right hand) and raise it just enough with the left hand to place the right hand underneath, so the edges of the palms and little fingers are touching. Slowly curl the fingertips upward slightly, and pull your hands gently toward you, until the fingertips catch just below the base of the skull, at the occipital ridge. Here they are in contact with several meridian points, including the gall bladder. This area is a major gathering point for tension.

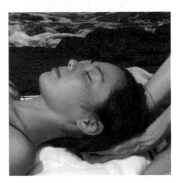

Position 4: Clavicle

Slowly uncurl the fingers and slip the hands forward with an outward-rotating motion, to free them from under the head. Now place them over the recipient's col-

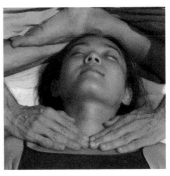

larbone (clavicle), fingertips meeting at the middle. The center of the clavicle is where several meridians connect, among them the stomach.

Position 5: Lower Ribs

Go around to the left side and place your hands gently over the bottom of the rib cage, fingertips of one hand meeting heel of the other at

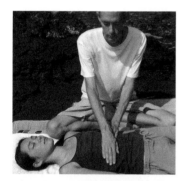

the tip of the sternum. This works the exit point of the liver meridian, which starts in the foot.

Position 6: Shoulders

Go back to the head of the table and ease your palms under the shoulders. Then curl the fingers slightly upward and pull back, almost locking the fingers into the shoulder blade. This area carries a great deal of energy to and from the head. The small intestine and gall bladder meridians pass through here.

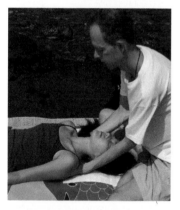

Position 7: Lower Back

Go around to the recipient's left side and very carefully push your left hand, palm up, under the back in the solar plexus area, with your palm under the spine. (It helps to ask them to raise their back a little.) Place your right hand on the person's left shoulder, as a comforting gesture. This position connects with the kidney-associated point on the bladder meridian—an important "water" point.

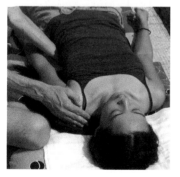

Revive the Recipient:

With your right hand on the recipient's left shoulder, cup your left hand slightly, just above and between the legs, and as near the feet as possible. In a swift motion, run your hand angling upward into the air, forward toward (and beyond) the recipient's head, extending the arm. At the same time give a short, sharp out-breath (forcefully whispering the sound of "Foo!"). The intent here is to reverse the energy flow, grounding and reviving the person. Tell them softly that the session is finished, and suggest that they remain lying down as long as they like.

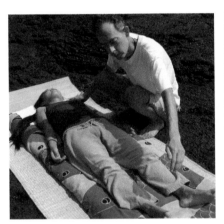 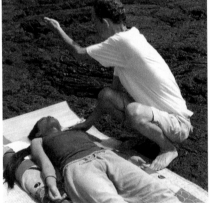

Twelve Positions

The following twelve hand positions have long been taught; in fact, many Reiki books refer to them as the "Basic Hand Positions," and I will list them only briefly here. Mr. Doi's *Modern Reiki Method for Healing* has some interesting comments on the effects of each position. There are four positions on the head, four on the front of the body, and four on the back.

Position 1: Face

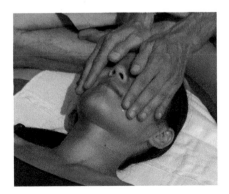

Position 2: Sides of head

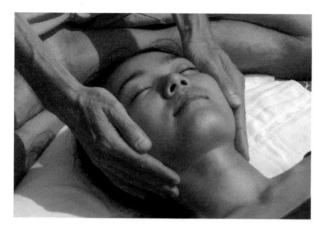

Position 3: Back of head

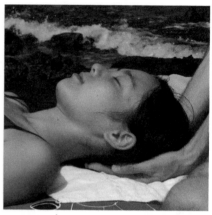

Position 4: Throat

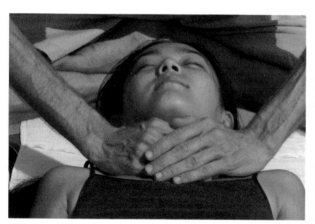

Position 5: Heart and thymus

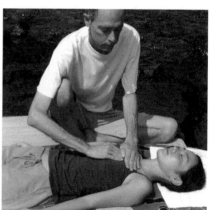

Position 6: Lower ribs

Position 7: Solar plexus

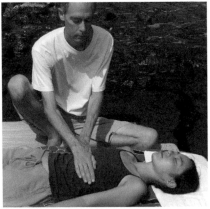

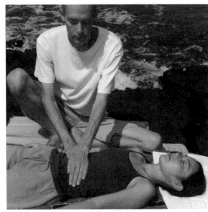

Position 8: Abdomen

Position 9: Shoulder blades

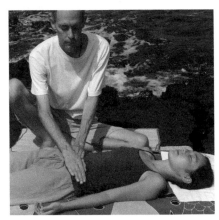

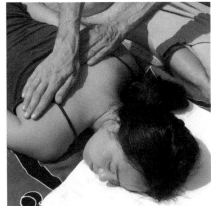

Position 10: Upper back   Position 11: Lower back   Position 12: Base of spine

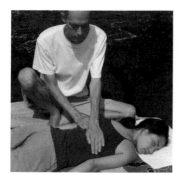 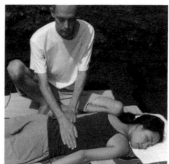 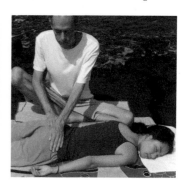

Seventeen Positions

In *The Spirit of Reiki*,[8] Walter Lübeck, a German Reiki teacher, gives a detailed description of this style of full-body treatment. Here, briefly, are the hand positions:

Position 1: Face   Position 2: Temples

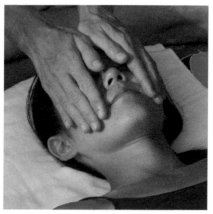 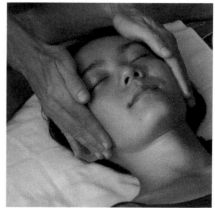

Position 3: Ears

Position 4: Back of head

Position 5: Throat

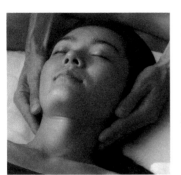
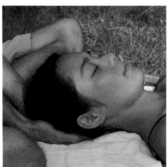
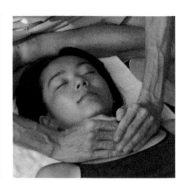

Position 6: Lower ribs, right side

Position 7: Lower ribs, left side

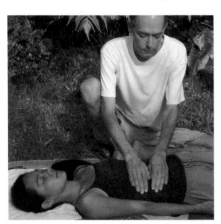
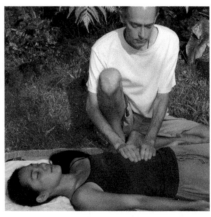

Position 8: Above & below navel

Position 9: Heart and thymus

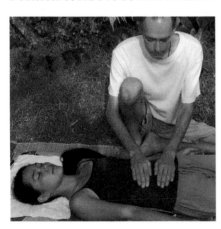
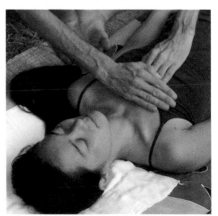

Position 10: Pelvis

Position 11: Tops of shoulders

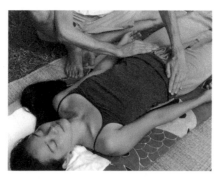

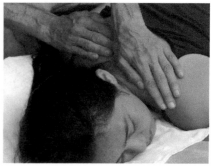

Position 12: Shoulder blades

Position 13: Lower ribs

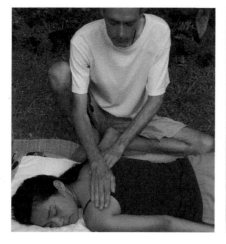

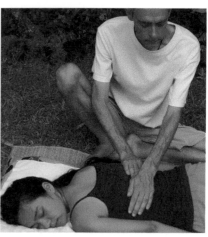

Position 14: Sacrum and tailbone

Position 15: Backs of knees

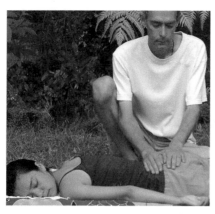

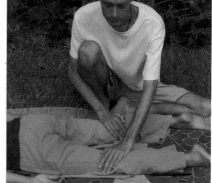

Position 16: Ankles

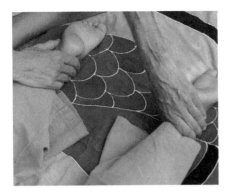

Position 17: Soles of feet

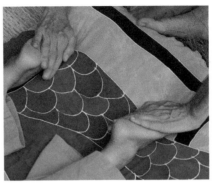

Treating Chakras via the Hands

Here's a way of treating the whole body, via the main chakras, by touching only the hands. This is not an Usui method, nor a Reiki method I've seen anywhere else. I learned the chakra connections from a Raja Yoga group and simply realized that they would make it possible to give Reiki to the whole body in this manner. It works because each of the seven major chakras is connected with a point on each of the hands, as shown here:

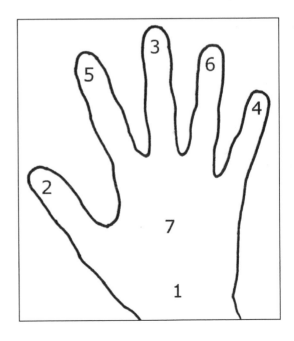

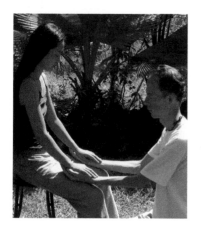

This treatment can be given with the recipient lying down, or sitting, or even standing. If the person is comfortable sitting, that may be the most convenient way. I sit facing the recipient, whose hands are held out toward me, palms down. I put my hands, palms up, under the recipient's. I start by giving Reiki simultaneously to the Crown (#7) and Root (#1) chakra points, in the palms. Then I take individual fingers in my hands, in the following sequence:

Ring fingers (connected to Brow Chakra, #6)
Index fingers (connected to Throat Chakra, #5)
Little fingers (connected to Heart Chakra, #4)
Middle fingers (connected to Solar Plexus Chakra, #3)
Thumbs (connected to Sacral Chakra, #2)

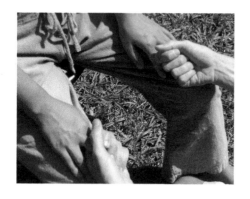

If time allows, I give at least five minutes of Reiki to each position, and finish by repeating the Crown (#7) and Root (#1) points in the palms. This is a remarkably effective, full-body treatment.

With the techniques in this chapter alone, you have the tools for healing yourself and others. You have the tools for healing everything, from a single chakra to the whole cosmos (and, remember, healing is nothing but "making whole," returning something to its original, perfect manifestation, its true Self). Even so, we'll look at more techniques in the next chapter—many of which have been traditionally used with Reiki in Japan.

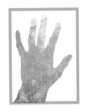

Chapter 4

Techniques and Training

"Traditional" Usui Techniques

In the Usui Gakkai, students are given a manual—the *Usui Reiki Hikkei*—purportedly written by Usui-sensei. The manual *(hikkei)* includes a Healing Guide *(shishin)*—an extensive list of hand positions for treating particular symptoms.[1] But actually these hand positions are the work of Dr. Hayashi.[2]

According to Hiroshi Doi, the following techniques were taught in Shoden by Usui-sensei:

Hand Positions

Doi-sensei seems to accept the Gakkai Healing Guide as indeed originating with Usui. In addition, he has said that the importance of treating the head was emphasized in all cases. I've seen slight variations taught as Usui's hand positions for the head. Treatments were given with the recipient seated. Here is one version:

1. One hand on forehead (hairline), the other on occiput
2. Temples
3. Upper back of head

4. Lower back of head and neck

5. Crown

(For illustration, see photos of head positions in "Sitting Treatment," Chapter 3.)

The following version comes from Usui's surviving students, via Chris Marsh and Taggart King. These students learned it in Shoden only for self-healing; treatment of others was not taught until Okuden. The wording here is from a manual by Taggart King:

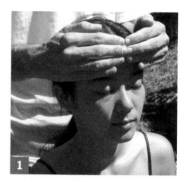

1: Front of forehead along the hairline, with your hands held with fingertips touching each other in the midline, and your palms facing towards you.

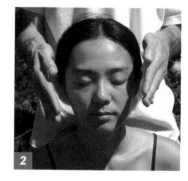

2: Hands hovering by the temples.

3: One hand at the back of the head, with the other hand resting on the forehead.

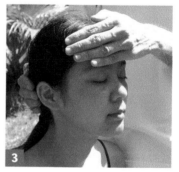

4: Both hands at the back of the neck/base of skull. The thumbs are joined from the tips to the base, and are pointing upwards. The rest of the palm and the fingers gently curve round the sides of the base of the skull/upper neck.

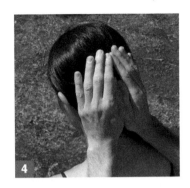

5: Rest both hands on the crown, overlapping one another.

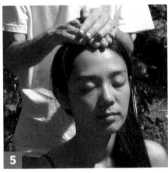

Taggart King notes that the first four positions are *mudras* (the Sanskrit word means "seal" or "mystery," and a mudra is a symbolic hand movement or body posture) from a Bodhisattva named Binzuru, renowned for healing abilities, and that using them invokes the healing powers of Binzuru.

In Shoden, students were taught to use these positions either by placing their physical hands on their own head or by imagining their own body sitting in front of them (facing the same direction), envisioning themselves placing their hands on it. Alternatively, the healing can be done merely by focusing one's attention at each position in sequence on the physical head, as though someone else were placing hands there.

Byosen Reikan-ho

In traditional Usui Reiki Ryoho, students are expected to become proficient in the technique of Byosen Reikan-ho. *Byosen* means "sick line" or "sick point," and *Reikan-ho* is a method of sensing the spirit of it. It's a technique, often called "scanning" in the West, for locating imbalance in the body. It's what was described already in the sitting treat-

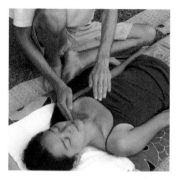 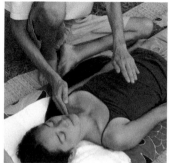 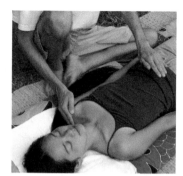

Byosen Reikan-ho in reclining treatment

ment: the feeling, in your hands, of notable sensations when sweeping the aura. Whether the recipient is sitting or reclining, bring your palms toward the body until you feel the aura, then sweep them gently down the length of the body, starting above the head and ending beyond the feet.

In a reclining treatment, if there is plenty of time, I like to treat the head and the front of the body thoroughly, and then scan to see if any rough spots remain. If so, give them Reiki (either in the aura, on the body, or both) until they feel smooth. Then smooth down the whole front of the aura, from head to feet as at the beginning. Treat the back thoroughly, do the same scanning procedure on it, and smooth down the whole back of the aura. Finish by smoothing up several times, from feet to head, to revive and energize. Let the person lie there and integrate the treatment until he or she feels ready to get up.

Using the *byosen* or "scanning" technique, we find imbalances and blockages in the aura, sometimes before any problem has manifested in the physical body. If we can heal them in the aura, we prevent them from becoming physical.

Reiji-ho

Reiji is the technique of positioning the hands by pure intuition, which can be accessed in whatever way is natural to each of us. The hands may simply feel where to go, or we may hear the message internally, or get it visually, or feel a sensation at the corresponding point in our own body. The important thing is to ask for inner direction, and then trust it in whatever form it comes to us. I believe this is really what Reiki is all about: connecting us to our more complete, more knowing, more authentic Self. It's about Self-discovery, which is the greatest empowerment of all, and what allows us to fulfill our life's purpose and to be most helpful to others.

When you first try these techniques, you may not feel much. But, if you keep practicing, your sensitivity will increase. In any case, it's good to give a full-body treatment as well.

At least two sources have said that the Usui Gakkai teaches the following as a typical model of an Usui Reiki treatment: First he would identify, via Reiji, the area where greatest healing was needed. There he would apply Reiki, usually with just one hand. The middle and ring fingers would be held together, extending forward, angling downward. They would be the main focal point for the energy—while the index finger and little finger were pointing forward horizontally. These and the thumb (which angled upward) were thought to disperse any "negative" energy.

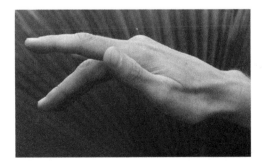

In this way, it was said, Usui would often give three-minute healings!

Nowadays, in the Gakkai version of this, only the thumb and little finger are used to disperse "negative" energy; the index finger is held together with the other two.

This certainly gives the rest of us something to work toward! Until we achieve that level of proficiency, it seems a good strategy to treat the head thoroughly—the entire body being represented in the head— and then to treat any particular spots on the body identified by Reiji or Byosen.

Nentatsu-ho

This is a technique for using Reiki to plant a message in the subconscious mind. (Mr. Doi cautions against confusing this with any method of healing with mind power.) It can be used (either for oneself or someone else) to change habitual behavior, to get the Reiki Concepts into the subconscious, to plant any kind of affirmation, etc. Obviously it should not be done without approval of the recipient, who determines what is to be affirmed.

When using affirmations, make sure they are stated positively—for example, "I eat only what is beneficial to me"; not "I don't eat junk food"—because the subconscious disregards negatives. (In the previous example, what it would hear and focus on is "junk food.") Also, state affirmations in the present, as statements of current reality. Don't say, "I will do ..." (which implies the future); say, "I do...." Don't say, "I want ..." (because the subconscious will perpetuate the lack of whatever you name); say, "I have ..." or "I am...."

The traditional way of doing this was merely to place the hands on the forehead, at the hairline, while transmitting the affirmation (either spoken aloud or silently in the mind). The affirmation can be repeated just a few times, or as long as desired.

There is a modern variation of this, which I like better. It uses one hand on the forehead and the other on the back of the head, at the top of the spine. I like to use my dominant hand on the forehead (sending from the conscious mind) and the other hand on the back (receiving in the subconscious mind). Then, after a few minutes of this, the affirmation is released and both hands are placed on the back of the head, giving Reiki there as long as desired.

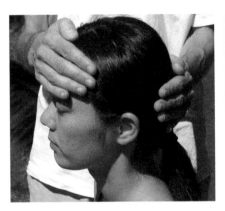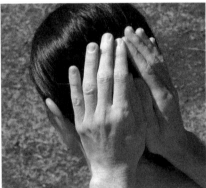

Nentatsu-ho, modern variation

Jakikiri Joka-ho

This is a technique for literally cutting off the existing energy flow to an object and energizing the object with Reiki instead. *This is to be used only on inanimate objects!*

If the object is small enough, hold it in the palm of your non-dominant hand. Relax and balance the body, take a breath down into the tanden, and hold it there. Now, with your dominant hand palm down, about two inches above the object, chop the air sharply, horizontally, three times—swinging the hand from near your body to beyond the fingertips of the other hand, ending each chop abruptly. Then breathe normally and give Reiki to the object with both hands for as long as desired.

If the object is too large for this, the procedure can be done at selected points, or a miniaturized mental image of the object can be used in the hand.

A modern variation of this includes an additional step: After applying the Reiki, the chopping procedure is repeated, to seal the Reiki in and keep other energies away.

Shuchu Reiki

Shuchu means "concentrated," and this is a way to increase the effectiveness of Reiki treatment. It's done by multiple people giving Reiki simultaneously to a recipient. This is especially beneficial in very difficult cases. It's believed that the effectiveness of the Reiki increases by the square of the number of givers. For example, with four people giving Reiki, the effect is sixteen times (four squared) as great as with one person giving.

Large numbers of people can be involved in this. If there are more givers than can actually put hands on the recipient, the extra ones put their hands on the backs of the primary givers (or on the backs of the secondary givers, if there are still more, etc.). I've seen groups doing this engulfed in actual clouds of heat waves! The Reiki is so powerful, some people say this should not be used on a recipient who is not emotionally stable. (Personally, I don't believe that Reiki will ever cause harm, no matter how it is applied; the recipient will not accept more of it than is beneficial.)

Renzoku Reiki

Renzoku means "marathon," and this is the procedure of two or more people taking turns giving Reiki to a recipient over a long period of time.

Reiki *Mawashi*

Mawashi means "current," and this is a way of passing a current of Reiki from person to person. The participants may sit or stand in a circle, either holding hands or with a small air space between hands. The left hand is customarily palm-up, the right hand palm-down. Reiki can be allowed to flow naturally, or can be deliberately sent in either direction around the circle.

Usui Shoden

Though Mr. Doi and the Gakkai seem to believe that the foregoing techniques were taught by Usui in Shoden (the first level of training), apparently most of them came from a Kiko manual published in 1927 by the Japanese Navy and issued to all Imperial Officers (and remember, the Gakkai was founded by some of these officers). Taggart King says that although Usui surely knew these techniques (from his own study of Kiko), they were not part of his method.

According to Usui's living students, Shoden was comprised of the following:

- receiving many Reiju empowerments
- chanting and living the Precepts
- practicing self-healing (including healing meditations)
- developing awareness of the hara/tanden and mindfulness (living totally in the present moment)
- studying selected waka (native poems; chosen because they contained kotodama, i.e., sacred sounds)
- practicing two energy exercises, Kenyoku and Joshin Kokkyu-ho (described below)
- no Reiki treatment of others

Kenyoku ("Dry bathing" or "Brushing off")

This is a method of cleaning one's energy or detaching from surrounding energies. It's done here in preparation for breathing-in spiritual Light. You can sit in a chair or in *seiza* (*sei* = proper, right, true; *za* = sitting posture) on the floor (see photo below).

1. Place the palm of the right hand on the upper left side of your chest, with fingertips in the indentation between where the collarbone and shoulder meet. The hand is lying flat on the chest.
2. Move the hand slowly in a straight line diagonally, to the right hip, where it stops. Breathe out as you make this movement.
3. Do the same with the left hand, starting on the right side and moving diagonally to the left hip, and breathing out again as you make the movement.[3]
4. Repeat steps 1 and 2.
5. Extend the left forearm straight in front of you, palm up, and place the right palm on the left wrist.
6. Brush the right palm across the length of the left hand and beyond the fingertips.[4] Breathe out as you make this movement.
7. Extend the right forearm, palm up, and brush across the hand with the left palm, in the same manner,[4] breathing out again.
8. Repeat steps 5 and 6.

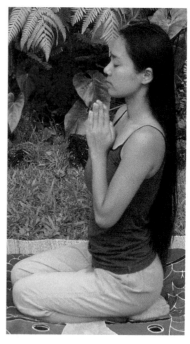

Seiza with gassho

Joshin Kokkyu-ho ("Purifying spirit Breathing method")

Kenyoku is followed immediately by Joshin Kokkyu-ho. This is also
done seated, in a chair or in seiza.

1. Rest the hands on legs, palms up and slightly cupped. Relax and
   breathe normally through the nose.
2. With the in-breath, visualize energy or golden-white light coming in on the breath and through the crown, pouring down
   through the body.
3. In the pause before exhaling, feel this light expanding instantly
   to fill the body, dissolving all tension.
4. With the out-breath, feel the light going out through the skin of
   the whole body, to infinity in all directions.

Usui's students were taught to practice these exercises every day, in
order to increase their vibrational rate and accelerate spiritual development, and to improve their capacity for transmitting Reiki.

Hatsurei-ho

In the Gakkai, a version of Kenyoku and Joshin Kokkyu-ho combined
is part of a longer sequence called Hatsurei-ho ("generating-spirit
method"), which comes from a Taoist Chi-gung movement. Students do
Hatsurei-ho and the teachers give them Reiju. According to Mr. Doi,
Usui-sensei taught Hatsurei-ho in the Okuden level of training, but this
is not confirmed by the surviving Usui students.

Many people find the daily practice of these exercises—either Usui's
Kenyoku and Joshin Kokkyu-ho or the Gakkai's Hatsurei-ho[5]—very
beneficial. You can practice them by yourself anytime. You may also

discover your own intuitive meditations, and they may change from time to time. I recommend using whatever technique works best, whatever feels most powerful and most authentic in your body at any time.

An Energy Exercise of My Own

The following exercise is one I have especially liked: my own combination of gassho and the Reiki Concepts, with kotodama and a breathing exercise.

First, a little background information about the elements of the exercise:

Gassho means "two hands coming together." This is a common posture for prayer in many cultures, if not universally. There is good reason for this: Bringing the palms of our hands together completes an electrical circuit in the body, and also balances each of the seven major chakras in the body (as we can see from the chakra connection-points in "Treating Chakras via the Hands"—see Chapter 3).

In Buddhist teaching, bringing the hands together is symbolic of the balancing of elements in the greater Universe:

Right hand—the Sun
Left hand—the Moon
Thumbs—the Void
Index fingers—Air
Middle fingers—Fire
Ring fingers—Water
Little fingers—Earth

Kotodama or *kototama* means "spirit words" or "spirit language"—fundamental sounds that carry creative power. This concept, like the practice of gassho, is common to many cultures around the world. The Christian Bible says it this way:

> "In the beginning was the Word,
> and the Word was with God,
> and the Word was God."
>
> (John 1:1 KJV)

A similar belief is expressed in Australian Aboriginal and Native American cultures, which tell of original beings who traversed the surface of the newborn Earth, singing the landscape into existence with magical songs.

In the ancient Shinto religion of Japan, kotodama were (and are) also used. Utilizing this Shinto understanding, Mikao Usui allegedly developed a set of kotodama to help his students connect with particular aspects within Reiki. (These are taught in the second and third levels, Okuden and Shinpiden—please see Note 20, Chapter 1, for more on this.)

One of the greatest authorities on kototama in recent times was an Aikido Master named Mikoto Masahilo Nakazono. The following is from his 1994 book *The Source of the Present Civilization:*

> The Kototama Principle was perfected 56,100 years ago. In that very ancient time, our ancestors grasped the reality of the entire universe as sound rhythm. The complete name of the principle of the fundamental life rhythms is Kototama Futomani.[6]

And, from Nakazono's 1984 publication *Inochi—The Book of Life:*[7]

> The Kototama Principle ... governs the activity of the life of the universe. It is the law of the operation of human capacity, its derivation, manifestation and action. ...

Some eight thousand years ago, the only true principle for human beings was hidden and civilization went its way in ignorance of it. . . .

The manifestation of human life, both body and spirit, is the activity of total human life in a priori universe:[8] Human = Universe. Human life is the universe itself; this explanation of our life is the basic premise of the Kototama Principle.

From *The Source of the Present Civilization:*

The content of the human capacities can be divided into five dimensions. The first is the source of the human physical constitution and its physical senses. To create the five senses of sight, hearing, smell, taste and touch, the a priori life rhythms pass through our a posteriori physical being, and meet the rhythms of our nervous system and brain.[9] This is happening at every second of our lives. Our nerves and brain are tuned to a permanent synchronization: their vibration changes in response to the incoming rhythms.[10]

From *Inochi:*

The first dimension's rhythm itself, of the life manifestation, comes out through the mouth as a sound. It comes out naturally as the sound of *U.* . . . [This sound rhymes with "blue."]

In this state of no name, no form, no number, phenomena of the total a priori universe manifest with the name or word of *U.* "In the beginning was the Word." (John, Chap. 1) refers to this word.[11]

Nakazono immersed himself for decades in the study and practice of the Kototama Principle. It is, like Reiki, a lifelong endeavor. I've just recently been introduced to Nakazono's books. At best, we might say, I have the tip of one little toe in the ocean of Kototama Principle. Even so—*and, clearly, taken out of context*—here are a few examples of kototama and their meanings or effects:

U (Oooo, rhymes with "blue")—the five physical senses

WU (Wooo)—capacity of the five physical senses

A (Ahhh, as in "ah")—spiritual action, the light of life

HA (Hahhh)—opening wider, expansion of the light of life

WA (Wahhh)—spiritual capacity

Now let's put the gassho and kototama together:

Sit or stand in the most balanced way. Bring the hands together and hold them wherever they feel most natural. For me, they often go immediately in front of the throat.

Take a natural breath, down into the tanden. When the breath is ready to come out, let it come out as a kototama, with the pitch as low as is comfortable. Make the sound of *A,* for instance. (See "How to Make the Sounds" in Chapter 7 for instructions on movement and positioning of the mouth; then just let the sound come out, as naturally and plainly as possible.)

You can make the sound of *A*—letting it flow as long as you like—and then follow it with the sound of *WA.* To make the *WA,* start with an *U* sound, which immediately becomes *WA* (U becoming double-U: *U-WA*). Feel the two sounds, *A* and *WA,* and the difference between them. With hands in gassho, while toning the kototama, you may also feel the different states of energy, from the Void, to Air, to Fire, to Water, to Earth. You can tone *A* and *WA* several times while focusing your awareness on the nature of each element (Void, Air, Fire, Water, Earth).

Then I like to follow this with a breathing exercise, incorporating the Reiki Concepts (in my own wording, plus one more).

This way of breathing, described below, is very good for balancing body energy and improving awareness. It's officially a yoga exercise, but I first learned it from a book called *The Law of the Rhythmic Breath* (by Ella Fletcher), which claimed this to be the original, natural pattern of human breathing. (Maybe that's why it seems to connect us more to our true nature.) It can be done standing, sitting, or lying on the back, with the spine straight and body relaxed. One cycle of breathing consists of the following:

Exhale, left nostril (close the right with a finger)
Inhale, left nostril
Exhale, right nostril (close the left with a finger)
Inhale, right nostril

Breathe down into the tanden, but not especially deeply. Just let the air move in and out naturally, without forcing it. The effects of this exercise are surprisingly powerful, and the breathing will become increasingly deep over time, naturally, with no attempt to make it happen.

One very easy way to do this exercise is in bed, before getting up in the morning, and again at night, before sleeping. You can also do it any time during the day, though I suggest not soon after eating. It is quite powerful, and five repetitions of the cycle are probably enough at any one time, at least until you've done the exercise regularly for a few weeks.

When you become familiar enough with the pattern that you're switching nostrils automatically, you can incorporate the following meditation (think these words in your mind as you breathe):

Cycle #1:

1. "I let go all fear and worry"[12] (feel these flying out, like a stream of birds, from the navel).
2. "I am Faith" (feel the Root Chakra as a basin of solid rock, which

is filled by the Sacral Chakra, a body of water: for instance, the Earth and the Sea).

3. "I let go all fear and worry" (same as 1 above).
4. "I am Faith" (same as 2 above).

Cycle #2:

1. "I let go all anger and frustration" (feel these flying out, like a stream of birds, from the navel).
2. "I am Peace; I welcome what IS" (feel this in the solar plexus, like the surface of a lake that's perfectly still, silent, reflective).
3. "I let go all anger and frustration" (same as 1 above).
4. "I am Peace; I welcome what IS" (same as 2 above).

Cycle #3:

1. "I give thanks" (extending out from the Heart Chakra).
2. "I am grateful" (taking All That Is into the Heart Chakra).
3. "I give thanks" (same as 1 above).
4. "I am grateful" (same as 2 above).

Cycle #4:

1. "I am kind to Self and others" (radiating out from the Throat Chakra).
2. "I am true to Source" (feel the Source energy welling up from Source-dimension[13] within the Throat Chakra).
3. "I am kind to Self and others" (same as 1 above).
4. "I am true to Source" (same as 2 above).

Cycle #5:

1. "I let go all sadness" (feel this flying out, like birds, from the Brow Chakra).

2. "I am Joy!" (imagine the feeling of angels!).

3. "I let go all sadness" (same as 1 above).

4. "I am Joy!" (same as 2 above).

After doing the exercise for some time, focusing on the *letting go* (of fear, anger, and sadness; in Cycles 1, 2, and 5), you may like to simplify those affirmations—using, respectively, just "I am Faith," "I am Peace," and "I am Joy!" I've made those changes, and a few others, resulting in the version below:

Cycle #1:

"I am Faith" (feeling the sprout of a green, growing, Tree element at the navel—going down through Water and Earth [Sacral and Root chakras] with the out-breath, coming up through Earth and Water [Root and Sacral chakras] with the in-breath).

Cycle #2:

"I am Peace" (feeling, in the solar plexus [third chakra], the element of Fire/Sun, radiating-out with the out-breath, and welling-up from within on the in-breath).

Cycle #3:

"I Do-without-doing, and gratefully" (feeling, in the lungs and heart [fourth chakra], the element of Air/Sky, radiating-out with the out-breath, and welling-up from within on the in-breath).

Cycle #4:

"I am Kind and True" (feeling, in the throat [fifth chakra], the total transparency of Ether/Truth, radiating-out with the out-breath, and welling-up from within on the in-breath).

Cycle #5:

"I am Joy!" (feeling, in the top of the head [sixth and seventh chakras], the golden-white light of Joy, radiating-out with the out-breath, and welling-up from within on the in-breath).

Then you may elect to repeat the gassho and kototama exercise (possibly using different kototama this time). Please let your own feelings guide you. I can't overemphasize that Reiki is about connecting to your true Self, to your innermost knowledge. Any techniques you learn from someone else are only starting points—and even the techniques you develop for yourself are merely tools. It's important not to invest them with powers they don't actually possess. I see them as "training wheels" or even, to some degree, "stage props." They are things we can use for as long as they feel right to us, but it's important to keep moving forward with the stream of our intuition as it leads us always to new and better things.

Selecting a Teacher

If you're already a Reiki person, I pray you're finding new and beneficial information, and inspiration, in this book. If you've not yet been initiated into Reiki, I greatly recommend it. Reiki has been, and continues to be, the foundation of my spiritual connection and practice. It brings me closer every day to realizing the real Self, closer to the unification of personal and Universal.

There are many "brands" of Reiki from which to choose, and countless Reiki teachers. As far as I know, the Reiki connection provided by Mikao Usui is the seed from which all other varieties have sprung. One of the most beautiful things about Reiki, to me, is that it truly is, as Usui envisioned, a "leaderless method." There are Reiki organizations that have created leaders and rules for themselves; but those of us who prefer to be independent are free to do so. Reiki is a supremely loving, inclusive, universal energy, which cannot be owned or controlled or legislated by any group or individual. The very nature of Reiki is to engender diversity and variety!

There's a very old saying, "When the student is ready, the teacher appears." That has certainly been my experience with Reiki: not once or twice or three times, but many. And, the times when I thought I was ready but really wasn't, nothing happened. So, the whole idea of "selecting" a teacher may be rather ludicrous. As with every experience in life, I believe our own vibrations draw to us the "right" teacher at the "right" time.

In case you're determined to seek out a teacher for yourself, or you find yourself trying to choose among more than one, or just as a way of confirming to yourself the "rightness" of a particular teacher, these questions may prove helpful:

Do I feel at ease in the presence of this person?

Is he or she happy to answer my questions, to tell me about Reiki, to let me experience it (and if so, how does it feel)?

How long has the person been practicing Reiki, how much training has he or she had (and from whom), and how much time was there between initiations into the different levels?

Does the person have an inclusive or an exclusive attitude? One of openness or secrecy? Is Reiki freely available or is it strictly priced?

There is no set of "right" answers to these questions. The important thing about the answers you receive is the feeling they give you in your body. In case you're still not sure what to do, look for signals in the environment. When the time is right for a certain action, it may be brought to your attention repeatedly; and when the time is not right, your attempts to bring it about are likely to fail or not to go smoothly.

As fast as Reiki is growing, still you may happen to live in a place physically remote from a teacher. Thanks to the instantaneous connection of Reiki itself, physical proximity is not required for empowerment; and verbal communication is quick and easy via email. Many teachers (myself included) offer remote empowerments and training.

Greatest blessings on your Reiki path!

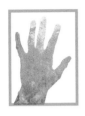

Chapter 5

Usui's Benevolence, and the Nature of Reiki

The Usui Memorial

At the grave of Mikao Usui is a large memorial stone, engraved with a story of his life and the beginning of his Reiho ("Spirit method"; also taken by some to be a shortened way of saying "Reiki Ryoho").

Thanks to James Deacon for allowing me to present this translation of the Memorial here. It can also be seen on his Web site—at www.aetw.org/reiki_usui_memorial.html. A printable PDF version is at www.aetw.org/reiki_pdf.htm.

In February, 1927, Usui-Sensei's students are said to have erected the memorial to his memory which now stands in a graveyard at the Jodo shu (Pure Land sect) Saihoji Temple, Tokyo.

Note that from the outset, the Memorial speaks of Usui-Sensei as the founder of Reiho (Spiritual Method), not Reiki.

REIHO CHOSO USUI SENSEI KUDOKU NO HI
Memorial of the Benevolence of Usui Sensei,
founder of Reiho (Spiritual Method)

English Version, Copyright © 2003 James Deacon
Translation (especially for AETW.org) by Jiro Kozuki

That which one attains within, as a result of disciplined study and training, is called Virtue, and that which can be offered to others by teaching, and methods of salvation is called Distinguished Service. Only the person of high merit and great virtue can be called a great founding teacher. Sages, philosophers, and brilliant men of old and the founders of new teachings and new religions were all like that. Usui Sensei can be counted among them. Usui Sensei developed the method that would improve mind and body by using the universal power. Having heard of his reputation, countless people from all over gathered and asked him to teach them the great way of the Spiritual Method, and to heal them.

His common name was Mikao and his other name was Gyoho (Kyoho). He was born in the village of Taniai in the Yamagata district of Gifu prefecture. His ancestor's name is Tsunetane Chiba. His father's name was Taneuji, and was commonly called Uzaemon. His mother's family name was Kawai.

Sensei was born in the first year of the Keio period, called Keio Gunnen (1865), on August 15th. He was a talented and hard working student; his ability was far superior to his fellows. When he had grown up, he travelled to Europe, America and China to study. He wanted to be successful in life, but couldn't achieve it. He worked hard but often he was unlucky and in need. However he didn't give up and he disciplined himself to study more and more.

One day he went to Kurama Yama to undergo rigourous spiritual discipline. On the beginning of the 21st day, suddenly he felt a large Reiki over his head. He attained an enlightenment and at that moment he comprehended the Spiritual Method. When he first used it on himself, it produced beneficial results immediately. After that, he tried it on his family. Since it was effective, he decided it was much better to share it with the public than to keep this knowledge solely for his own family. He opened a training centre[1] in Harajuku, Aoyama, Tokyo to teach and practice the Spiritual Method in April of the 11th year of the Taisho period (1922).

Many people came from far and wide and asked for the guidance and therapy, and even lined up outside of the building.

In September of the twelfth year of the Taisho period (1923), there was a devastating earthquake. Everywhere there were groans of pain from the injured. Usui Sensei felt pity for the people, and took the Spiritual Method into the devastated city and used its healing powers on the survivors, curing and saving innumerable people.

This is just a broad outline of his relief activities during such an emergency.

Later on, his training centre became too small. In February of the 14th year of Taisho (1925 A.D.) he moved to a new training centre in Nakano, outside Tokyo. Due to his increased fame he was often invited to many places. Sensei, accepting the invitations, went to Kure and then to Hiroshima and Saga, and reached Fukuyama. It was during his stay in Fukuyama that unexpectedly he became ill and died, aged 62.* It was March 9 of the 15th year of Taisho (1926 A.D.)

[*NOTE: According to the dates given, Usui-Sensei would have actually been 60 at the time of his death. However, apparently there is an ancient Japanese tradition that a child is considered to be 'one' at birth, and is seen as being a year older at each new year, rather than the birthday that falls in that year. An alternative explanation for the discrepancy could have something to do with the fact that, at the time of Usui Sensei's birth, Japan used a different calendrical system. The change over to the 'western' system in 1873 may have led to mistakes in the recording of exact dates of events in the immediately preceding years.]

His wife was named Sadako, from the Suzuki family. A boy and a girl were born. The boy's name was Fuji who carried on the Usui family after his father's death. Sensei was mild, gentle and modest by nature and he never behaved ostentatiously. His was physically big and strong. He always had a contented smile. However, in the face of adversity, he sought a solution with determination and patience. He had many talents and liked to read, and his knowledge of history, medicine, psychology, divination, incantation, physiognomy and Buddhist scriptures was great.

On reflection, the Spiritual Method not only cures diseases, but also balances the spirit and makes the body healthy using innate healing abilities, and so, helps achieve happiness.

So, when it comes to teaching, first let the student understand the Meiji Emperor's admonitions; and let them chant the Five Precepts mornings and evenings, and keep them in mind:

Firstly: Don't get angry today, Secondly: Don't worry today, Thirdly: Be grateful today, Fourthly: Work diligently today, Fifthly: Be kind to others today.

These are truly great teachings for cultivation and discipline in keeping with those great teachings of the ancient sages and the wisemen. Sensei named these teachings 'the Secret Method of Inviting Blessings' and 'the Spiritual Medicine to cure many diseases.' Notice the outstanding features of the teachings. Furthermore, when it comes to teaching, it should be as simple as possible and not difficult to understand. It is important to start from a place close to you. Another noted feature is that while sitting in silent meditation with your hands held in prayer and reciting the Five Precepts, a pure and healthy mind will be cultivated. Its true value is in daily practice. This is the reason why the Spiritual Method became so popular.

Recently the state of the world has altered and people's thoughts have changed a great deal. Hopefully, the spread of this Spiritual Method will be of great help to people who have a confused mind or who do not have morality. Surely it is not only of benefit in curing chronic diseases and lingering complaints?

The number of students of Sensei's teaching is already over 2,000. Among them, senior students who remained in Tokyo are maintaining Sensei's training centre, and others in different provinces also are trying to spread the Spiritual Method as much as possible. Although Sensei died, the Spiritual Method will continue to spread far and wide. Ah, what a great thing Sensei has done, to have shared this Spiritual Method with the people out there after having been enlightened within!

Lately, many students came together and decided to erect this memorial in the graveyard at Saihoji Temple in the Toyotama district to honour his benevolence, and to spread the Spiritual Method to the people in the future. I was asked to write these words. As I deeply appreciate his work and am pleased with the very friendly teacher-disciple relationships among fellow students, I could not refuse the request, and I wrote this summary in the hope that people will be reminded to look up to him with reverence.

Composed by: Masayuki Okada, Doctor of Literature—subordinate 3rd rank, 3rd Order of Merit.

Calligraphy by: Navy Rear Admiral Juzaburo Ushida—subordinate 4th rank, 3rd Order of Merit, distinguished service 4th class.

February, the 2nd year of Showa (1927 A.D.)

Ki, the Energy of Life

Ki is the Japanese word meaning, generally, the energy of life. Within this ki, a hierarchy of seven particular energies has been distinguished, as follows:[2]

Kekki—the ki of blood—provides fundamental strength. It is the most powerful and most basic of the seven energies, and the least structured. Associated with the Root Chakra.

Shioke—the ki of salt or minerals—provides bodily structure and connectedness, which makes possible and organizes to a degree the action of Kekki. Also associated with the Root Chakra.

Mizuke—the ki of water or liquids—makes possible relationship and communication (by allowing the flow of Kekki among various forms of Shioke). It is the basic energy of all emotions, allowing for nourishment and metabolism. Associated with the Sacral Chakra.

Kuki—the ki of air or gases—provides the motivation for self-discovery. It gives us the ability to define our own course in life, not to be overly influenced by others. Also, the energy of digestion (of ideas as well as physical food). Associated with the Solar Plexus Chakra.

Denki—the ki of "thunder"—gives the ability to balance our own ego with consideration for others. The element of Thunder implies the forces of Heaven—and Denki makes possible our trust in a Divine Creator, as well as feelings of love, empathy, fairness, tolerance, and understanding toward our fellow beings. Associated with the Heart Chakra.

Jiki—"magnetic power" or "gathering force"—provides charisma and aligns us with our true, Divine will. It gives the qualities of truth, beauty, and kindness. It attracts the perfect complement to our own being in every situation, as well as coordinating the five lower energies. Associated with the Throat Chakra.

Reiki—"soul force" or "spiritual power"—organizes and directs all the lower energies in the most holistic, synergistic way. In the material world, this is the energy closest to the Divine Creator, the Source of all energy and life. Reiki is associated with the Brow Chakra, and acts as a bridge between the material energies and the purely spiritual energy, called Shinki, from which everything is created and to which everything eventually returns.

These seven energies are also listed by Michio Kushi in *Macrobiotic Home Remedies*. Kushi translates **REI KI** as "ki of spirit," and "the invisible force of soul." He explains further:

All of these stages of *ki* came out from **SHIN KI**, God-*ki*. Out of *Shin Ki* (the source), *Rei Ki* (yin and yang) is born. Between yin and yang, *Ji Ki* (magnetism) arises, and next vibration, in the form of electricity *(Den Ki),* is produced. Then atmosphere, water and minerals are formed. We take all these in the form of food and transform them into *Kek-ki, ki* of blood, which nourishes our body.[3]

Even so, is there only one Reiki, or is Reiki a different energy for each individual? To me, the individual variation seems undeniable. Reiki, received through different people, feels different, even though there are fundamental similarities. From the Japanese understanding of seven bodily energies, presented above, we can say that Reiki is the "highest" of those energies. But one person's highest energy is very likely different than another person's highest energy.

Rick Rivard (a well-known Reiki teacher in Vancouver, who helped organize and hosted the first URRI conference there) talks about the idea of highest energy. He opines that Reiki empowerment/attunement is an attempt to connect the recipient to the highest energy (Reiki) of Mikao Usui. He says that, through the use of spirit guides, he has connected people to their own "highest healing energy"—which they felt to be different and more powerful than Reiki (to which they were already connected).[4] He also believes that the various flavors of Reiki, which have arisen since Usui, are merely the highest energies of their personal creators. But it seems to me self-evident that Reiki is indeed each person's own highest energy. Also, even though my Reiki (highest energy) is different than your Reiki (highest energy), they both connect us to the Source of All That Is!

Here's something relevant, from Dave King:[5]

In the mid 1990s my associate Shen Lissa (Melissa Riggall) stayed for a month with Tatsumi-san who was a student of Chuujirou Hayashi from 1927 to 1931. One day she pointed to a photo of the Usui concepts in Tatsumi-san's house. She noted the term "Reiki" and said that this was how the West referred to the hand healing system. Tatsumi-san said that the hand healing was simply referred to as te-áte, and that by using the term "reiki," O-Sensei (Usui Sensei) had been referring to his ancestors. **Usui Reiki Ryoho** simply means 'Usui system **for connecting with your ancestral self'**—something that is already within each one of us from the moment of conception.

And this, from Taggart King, on the subject of Reiju, Usui's empowerment procedure:

> The empowerment kotodama represented creative energy, regenerative energy, the energy of rebirth. The idea here is that when Reiju is carried out it connects the recipient to the energy, allowing them to be 'reborn': reborn in the sense of creating a place within that is 'what we originally were,' the state within the ovum when we were Divine essence in complete connection to the universe. The energy was the essence of earth and heavenly energy, white light, source, ultimate being.[6]

This confirms my own feeling that Reiki is connecting me to my true, original Self. Taggart's description seems to go beyond the ancestral connection, while also including it (by referring to the fertilized ovum in the womb).

Again, it seems to me that Usui's method connects us not to Usui's highest energy but to our own highest energy; to our own ancestral and Source energy, to our real Self.

The idea of such a connection between the personal self and a greater Self (sometimes perceived as the Soul, or a Guardian Angel, Guardian Spirit, or even a God) appears in many cultures and teachings. In Hawai'i the ancient tradition of spiritual understanding has come to be called Huna. It's generally accepted that many of its secrets (the word *Huna* itself means "secret") have been lost, though various researchers have attempted to reconstruct and understand the ancient teachings as much as possible.

One of the best known of these researchers was Max Freedom Long—known especially for his books *The Secret Science Behind Miracles* (1948) and *The Secret Science at Work: The Huna Method as a Way of Life* (1953).[7] Max described the Huna understanding of a human being as comprised of three individual spirits, which he called the "low self," "middle self," and "High Self." The "low self," he said, was the childlike one, in charge of the physical and auric bodies, and of memory; the "middle self"—"the one who speaks"—was the rational (more or less!) being that we most often think of as our self; and the "High Self" was comparable to what many people would call a Guardian Angel. The "High Self" was completely separate from the "middle self," and connected to the "low self" only by an auric cord. This cord extended, apparently without limit, allowing the "High Self" to be either very near the physical body or at any distance from it, at any given moment.

Long attempted to discover how the ancient *Kahunas* ("Keepers of the secrets") had accomplished miraculous things through prayer (the last real Kahuna having passed away hundreds of years previously). He came to believe that the process involved the "middle self" communicating its desire, telepathically, to the "low self"; then the "low self" passing on this request to the "High Self," via the auric cord connecting the two. "As for the High Self," he said, "*which has no limitations* [emphasis mine] except as imposed by the low and middle selves through failing to do their part, we will find practical proof of its powers, once we have learned to make and sustain working contact with it."[8]

To me, this "High Self" sounds very much like what Reiki connects us to; and Long's description of the auric cord brings to mind immediately my own feeling of Reiki as an "extension cord" to my real Self. His perception of the Huna prayer procedure is strikingly similar to the procedure of doing Reiki: We get the rational "middle self" out of the picture for a while and let the childlike "low self" connect with the unlimited "High Self"—and miraculous things tend to happen!

There is corroboration of this general theme also in Johrei ("purifying spirit"), where it's taught that we are each watched over by a higher self, called the Yukon, who exists in the spirit world and is always connected to us, and to whom we can (very beneficially) send Johrei energy.

Part Two
The Deep Inside (Okuden)

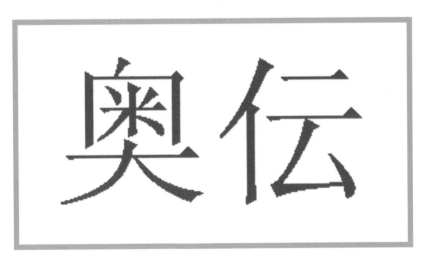

Kanji image courtesy Dave King

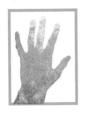

Chapter 6

Usui Sensei, Usui Society

Usui's Okuden

Living students of Mikao Usui in Japan say that their Okuden (second-level) training consisted of the following:

- receiving Reiju (repeatedly)
- practicing daily energy exercises
- studying Buddhist Sutras (Lotus, Heart, Diamond)
- continued attention on developing mindfulness

Within Okuden were two levels. Students in Okuden Zenki (the first level):

- developed their abilities to become "Earth energy" and "Heaven energy" (through daily work with specific meditations and/or kotodama)
- practiced giving Reiki to others (though this was not a major focus)

Students in Okuden Kuki (the second level) learned to connect with other beings by realizing the Oneness of all life (through daily work with a specific meditation and/or kotodama).

It was common for a student to work as long as nine months at realizing each of the energies, Earth and Heaven, and the consciousness of Oneness. Each energy was taught separately: Only when the student had learned Earth energy sufficiently was Heaven energy introduced; and only when Heaven energy was mastered would Oneness be introduced (which was seen not as an energy *per se,* but a state of mind).

It's unlikely that a student would have practiced "distant healing" as done today. The focus was on Self, and on realizing that actually there is *no* distance, only Oneness. Also, Taggart King points out that not every student would necessarily go beyond Okuden Zenki. It was very much a step-by-step process.

The Gakkai's Okuden

In the Usui Reiki Ryoho Gakkai, Okuden is also divided into Zenki and Kuki. Beyond that, there are many differences from what some of Usui's students learned as Okuden.

Zenki

According to Hiroshi Doi, Okuden Zenki in the Gakkai has traditionally included the following:

- *Hatsurei-ho*

  This is an exercise for "generating Spirit"—increasing one's capacity for Reiki. As I learned it from Mr. Doi, it consisted of Kenyoku followed immediately by Joshin Kokkyu-ho (see descriptions of these in "Usui Shoden," Chapter 4), plus a final bit of breathing and visualization. That was—while holding the hands in gassho— simply visualizing/feeling (on the in-breath) the light of Reiki coming into the hands and going to the hara; then visualizing/feeling (on the out-breath) the light of Reiki going from hara to hands, and radiating out from there.

- *Uchite Chiryo-ho*

  This (in addition to Reiki) is patting the body with hands, particularly for areas of numbness.

- *Oshite Chiryo-ho*

  This (in addition to Reiki) is pushing with fingertips or thumbs, particularly for areas of stiffness.

- *Nadete Chiryo-ho*

  This (in addition to Reiki) is stroking the body with hands to help increase the energy flow, usually stroking from top to bottom and/or from left and right toward the center.

- *Koki-ho and Gyoshi-ho*

  These are, respectively, giving Reiki through the breath and through gazing with the eyes. In Koki-ho, the out-breath is from the mouth, gently, with lips pursed. Gyoshi-ho is directing Reiki with a soft, unfocused gaze.

As with the "traditional" Usui techniques presented in Chapter 4, Taggart King says that these seem to have come from the Japanese Navy's 1927 Kiko manual—and were very likely never taught by Usui. Also, Taggart's version of Uchite, Oshite, and Nadete are performed in the aura, not on the physical body—as follows:[1]

Uchite:

This means to lightly and rhythmically tap or pat the chi field with either your palm or fingertips. This is useful to relieve stagnation or congestion and to improve circulation. In Tui-na Chinese Massage, tapping is applied directly to the body for the same purpose and the therapist taps with the fingers, the palm, or the back or side of the hand or fist, to produce varying degrees of stimulation.

In terms of the five elements,[2] tapping the chi field represents Water, and the movements are seen as causing any stuck energy to disperse into the underlying tissues, like water finding the lowest level.

Oshite:

This means to ever so slightly open and close the palm. Stretch the fingers and hand open, then relax. Do this repeatedly at a steady pace. The chi is emitted from the centre of the hand. The indications for pulsing are similar to tapping. It stimulates and improves circulation. Pulsing can be used over any area of the body that requires it, including specific acupuncture points. If you pulse directly over a point, it is claimed to be easy to feel tingling and warmth at that point, or radiating along the associated meridian.

Nadete:

This is very useful for congestion or pain. The fingertips sweep down the patient's energy field, as though brushing the pain away.

In terms of the five elements, side-to-side or circular movements represent Earth and are designed to be soothing and reassuring.

Here is Taggart's description of Koki-ho and Gyoshi-ho:

These techniques of sending Reiki using the eyes and the breath demonstrate the importance of intent. If you intend that Reiki travels with your gaze then it does so, and the energy takes on some of the characteristics of looking in terms of being focused, precise and piercing. If you intend that Reiki travels with your breath, it does so, and takes on some of the characteristics of breath in terms of working superficially and flitting rapidly from where it was sent to where it was needed.

The benefit of conveying energy with the eyes or breath as well as the hands is that you can "touch more bases" at one time. You can direct the energy with your hands into two locations, and direct it to a third place using the eyes or the breath. Alternatively, you can intensify the Reiki effect in one place by using two hands, and your breath or your eyes. Using the eyes or breath to convey the energy means that you can direct Reiki to places where it would be inappropriate to touch.

Petter [author of *Reiki Fire* and other books] says that the key to directing Reiki with the eyes seems to be to defocus the eyes, to look with soft focus, to look through the area where we want to send the energy, and to intend that the energy travels with your gaze. He says that you should look "with a loving state of being" behind you.

This technique can be used with photographs as a way of sending distant healing, by staring through a photograph...

The technique can be used in conjunction with the Reiki symbols, by visualising [them] over the targeted area, for example.

The instructions for sending Reiki with your breath are as follows: place the tip of your tongue on the roof of your mouth and inhale. As you inhale, draw down energy through your crown, and as you exhale onto your client, be conscious of energy flowing with the breath. You do not need to blow a hurricane, and the recipient does not even have to feel the movement of air for the technique to work. What is important is your intention that Reiki is transmitted with your breath.

It is also possible to use this technique in conjunction with the Reiki symbols: as you inhale, draw one of the Reiki symbols on the roof of your mouth with your tongue (practice!). Leave the tip of your tongue on the roof of your mouth, as before. Exhale as before onto your client. It would also work just to visualise the Reiki symbol on the roof of your mouth, of course.

Arjava Petter suggests that you can use this technique as a form of distant healing, by blowing at a photograph. . . .

Mr. Doi has also described two other Gakkai techniques, Heso Chiryo-ho and Tanden Chiryo-ho.

Heso Chiryo-ho

This is based on the importance of the navel *(heso).* We were connected via the navel with our mother while in the womb—and we can use the navel as a connection point with the greater Universe. This "treatment" is merely putting fingertips—of the middle and fourth fingers and the thumb, of one hand—into the navel together; directing Reiki there, feeling the pulse; maybe also feeling a cosmic umbilical connection there, bringing our personal vibration into harmony with that of Universal Spirit.

Tanden Chiryo-ho

This is a method for stimulating the removal of toxins from the body, by directing Reiki to the tanden. One hand is placed on the tanden, the other on the forehead, at the hairline. While feeling the Reiki at the forehead, the body is given an instruction to detoxify (similar to the giving of an affirmation in traditional Nentatsu-ho; see Chapter 4). This is done as long as desired, then both hands are placed on the tanden, directing Reiki there.

Kuki

As traditionally taught in the Usui Gakkai, Mr. Doi has described Oku-den Kuki as including the following:

- The receiving of three symbols
- *Seiheki Chiryo-ho* (mental technique)

    This is the same as the modern version of Nentatsu-ho (see "'Traditional' Usui Techniques" in Chapter 4) except, at the end, only one hand is on the back of the head.

- *Hanshin Koketsu-ho* (half-body blood cleansing)

    For this, it's customary (and most functional) to remove the recipient's clothing above the waist. *However, that may be a risky thing to do, depending on local laws and how well you know the recipient. In many places, it is illegal to ask a recipient to remove clothing unless you are a licensed massage therapist or medical doctor.*

    The procedure is—with recipient lying on stomach—to sweep the palms of your hands down the recipient's back, starting at the base of the neck, sweeping the palms outward, to left and right, as they go downward. This is done maybe ten to fifteen times. Then, holding the index and middle fingers of each hand together, those two fingers of the left hand are placed on the left side of the spine (at base of neck); the corresponding fingers of the right hand are placed on the right side of the spine (at base of neck); then both sets of fingertips are swept together down the length of the spine. To me, it seems natural to do this while breathing out (either through the nose or mouth; and maybe as a hado breath—see Chapter 4, Note 3). The fingertips come to rest, two on each side of the tailbone. They stay there through the out-breath and while the breath is paused for a moment before the next in-breath. Like the sweeping-down of the palms, this sweeping-and-holding movement of the fingers is repeated ten to fifteen times.

From Taggart King:

Running down the back are the Bladder, Gall Bladder and Governing Vessel meridians, and moving the hand(s) along the back in the way described above would have the effect of stimulating these. The Bladder meridian in particular is very good at dispersing energy. There are also special acupuncture points along the length of the back, and the hand movements would direct Reiki into every meridian, stimulating them and in effect "touching lots of bases" at the same time. Various branches of the sympathetic nervous system emerge from between the vertebrae on either side of the spine, so they would be affected by your actions too.

The Blood Exchange can be seen as a way of encouraging the body to detox, and can be used routinely at the end of a Reiki treatment, for example. It seems to help people to "come round" and feel clear-headed at the end of a treatment.

Also in the Gakkai version of Okuden Kuki is:

* *Zenshin Koketsu-ho* (full-body blood cleansing)

  This begins by giving Reiki to the head (front, back, sides, fore-head, and base of skull in back); then to lungs, heart, stomach, and intestines. Then the palms of both hands, together, are used to sweep the length of each arm of the recipient, from shoulder to fin-gertips, several times. The same sweeping motion is done (again, several times) from hips/thighs to the tips of the feet.

In a manual given to students in the Gakkai, Usui is quoted as mentioning some of these techniques. However, Chris Marsh has said that the manual appears to have been "edited" (and the techniques taken from a 1927 Kiko manual).

- *Enkaku Chiryo-ho* (distant healing)

  Traditionally, in the Gakkai, Okuden Kuki also includes Enkaku Chiryo-ho ("distant" healing). This is taught using three of the four Reiki symbols. The symbols were not part of Mikao Usui's revelation on Mount Kurama (as told by Hawayo Takata). They were borrowed from Chinese Buddhism, late in Usui's life, as an aid for certain students. They were taught to Dr. Hayashi and his fellow navy men Ushida and Taketomi—and to one of the surviving students of Usui known to Chris Marsh.

  Arjava Petter says that Usui taught distant healing by using a photograph. It's not certain, however, that distant healing was even taught overtly to many students. It was an ability that would naturally suggest itself when the student began to realize a state of Oneness with other beings; and the emphasis of Usui's teaching was on self-healing and spiritual awakening.

Emails from Dave King

Dave King was introduced to both Usui-do (a spiritual practice) and Eguchi Te-no-hira Ryoji (a religion based on healing, developed by Usui's close friend and student Toshihiro Eguchi) in 1971 in Morocco, by a student of Eguchi, Yuji Onuki. Since then Dave has made various trips to Japan, learning from students of both Usui and Hayashi. He has greatly improved my understanding of conditions and events in

Japan during Usui's time, and of some of Usui's original teachings and the ways in which they came to be transformed. The following insights are taken from his correspondence with me (2002–2005):

On the difference between Gakkai and Kenkyukai:

Gakkai implies an association for educational purposes. It is often used for groups of academics or clerics. The term can also be used for clubs.

Kenkyukai implies an association for research purposes. One was able to do "research" into healing systems as a "front" to a religious activity. Both Hayashi and Eguchi chose this route; they were genuinely doing research and both published papers.

On the proliferation of new religions in Usui's time:

Most religions were quite small and were formed as societies and associations by those who felt at a loss due to the domestic conditions caused by the opening up of the country to foreign trade but were not satisfied with the rigidity of state Shinto.

Christianity had influenced many Japanese religions of the time but the offering of wine and wafers (sacrament) was replaced with an offering of divine energy (reijuu)....

It is clear from discussions with several still-living students of Usui, Hayashi and Eguchi (which includes the nun Suzuki that is in communication with Chris Marsh) that there were several versions of Usui's system and none of them were gakkai (most were kenkyukai). It is most likely that the URR Gakkai was created by the rear admirals after Usui's death and is based on Usui's system as it was in 1926.

What has NOT been made clear to the Western public is that the versions of Usui's systems that came into being in late 1925 and early 1926 were religions. The 1926 system met the requirements of current legislation regarding religions based on healing simply by dedicating each meeting to Meiji (Although Meiji had been dead since 1912 he was still considered divine and reading his poems would have reduced the chance of prosecution for Lésé Majesté—a capital offense[3]).

The URR Gakkai is clearly a religious society. The opening activities, including Kenyoko-hou and reijuu, are typical of post-restoration healing religions. The chanting of Meiji's poems appears to have been added to keep the whole thing legal. The Bureau of Shrines and Temples of the Home Ministry had the task of policing new religions and spiritual groups under the strict laws enacted in the reign of Meiji and Taisho.

I [Dave King] do not believe that ANY of this Gakkai material was ever practiced by Usui.

- Tatsumi had no knowledge of it. Hayashi kept true to Usui's pre-1925 teachings until 1931.
- In November 1923, when Eguchi began to teach his own system in Usui's dojo, Usui would not permit Eguchi to offer prayers. We had this from both Mariko-Obaasan and Onuki. Eguchi went on to teach thousands of students his system at Nishida's Ittoen Center … The "Usui Hikkei" is actually parts of Eguchi's manual with added Meiji poems in a new front cover! Usui-Do is experiential and can not be described in a handout or guidebook and none of my teachers are aware of any handouts by Usui.
- Mariko-Obaasan told us that activities of a religious nature began to be incorporated into the dojo in late 1925. (The rear admirals took over the dojo in November 1925 but Hayashi had joined in May of the same year.) This must have been the start of the URR Gakkai. Of course later members of the Gakkai would not have known what had happened in Usui's dojo before the arrival of the rear admirals thus the assumption by Hiroshi Doi that these activities were part of Usui's system.

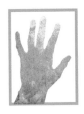

Chapter 7

Symbols and *Kotodama*

The Inner Aspects

We're now learning that Usui-sensei identified an Earth energy, a Heaven energy, and a state of mind or being called Oneness. These are what he taught as "the deep inside" of Reiki, according to some of his living students. Most of his students learned to "become" Earth and Heaven and Oneness through daily meditations and/or kotodama. Dr. Hayashi was taught symbols instead, which he then taught Hawayo Takata. From her, the symbols went around the world, and they have defined the world's perception of Reiki until very recently.

Even in Japan, in the Usui Gakkai, the symbols are what have been taught. This makes perfect sense, now that we've learned how the Gakkai was actually started by Usui's final students—Hayashi, Taketomi, and Ushida—who were taught symbols instead of kotodama or meditations. This fact in itself—that the Gakkai seems to have no knowledge of Usui's meditations or kotodama—appears to confirm that Usui himself did not start the Usui Gakkai.

Reiki Symbols

We know of four symbols taught by Usui, three of them in Okuden. The names of the Okuden symbols are:

Cho Ku Rei (also called the Focus or Power symbol)

Sei He Ki (also called the Harmony symbol)

Hon Sha Ze Sho Nen (also called the Connection or Distance symbol)

Here, in table form, is a summary of qualities associated with these symbols by some of Usui's living students:

■ **Table 7.1**

Okuden symbols and their qualities

#1 Focus Cho Ku Rei	#2 Harmony Sei He Ki	#3 Connection Hon Sha Ze Sho Nen
Earth energy	Heaven energy	
Heavy, grounding, strengthening (body and mind)	Light, etheric	
	Intuition, psychic awareness	State of being Oneness
Physical healing		
	Mental focus	
Forest green in color	Golden in color	

There is evidence to suggest that what Usui taught the naval officers about "the deep inside" was different than what he taught others. Not only did he give them symbols, but the symbols may have had different associations than what he previously taught. The navy men were his final students, and the change may simply indicate an evolution in Usui's understanding.

Tatsumi's Version

Reiki teacher Dave King studied with a student of Hayashi, a Mr. Tatsumi, who claimed that Hayashi taught him exactly what he had learned from Usui. Tatsumi passed these teachings on to Dave King, who suggests that the Okuden symbols have origins in a group of three Buddhist deities known as the Amida Sanzon. He says in an email: "In Tatsumi's notes were detailed descriptions of the origins and use of all four symbols. There were several references to Taoist documents such as the Tao Zang as well as mentioning the Amida Sanzon link."

These three deities and their correlations with the Okuden symbols, according to Dave King, are tabulated below:

■ **Table 7.2**

Okuden symbols related to Amida Sanzon deities

Reiki Symbol	Buddhist Symbol	Deity	Celestial Body
#1 / Focus	Power	Seishi	Earth
#2 / Harmony	Light	Amida	Sun
#3 / Connection	Love	Kannon	Moon

King makes a point of referring to the symbols either by number or as Focus, Harmony, and Connection; he says that in Japan they are never called Cho Ku Rei, Sei He Ki, and Hon Sha Ze Sho Nen. This is to avoid confusion, since the written symbols are not the same as the written kanji for those Japanese words.

Apparently, at some point, Usui's thinking evolved from the Taoist model (Earth-Heaven-Man) to the Amida Sanzon trinity (the Buddhist deities Seishi-Amida-Kannon). Dave King makes the above associations among the deities, the symbols, and the celestial bodies—but he states emphatically that the symbols do not *represent* Earth and Sun and Moon. He explains it this way:

- that Cho Ku Rei represents (or is represented by) Seishi
- that Earth represents (or is represented by) Seishi
- that Cho Ku Rei DOES NOT represent (nor is it represented by) Earth.

Still, all three (deity, symbol, and celestial body) are clearly associated in some way.

Dave King also says:

I do not believe that the symbols have "energies" in the way that is taught in the West. Reverend Takata appears to have mapped Hayashi Reiki Ryoho Kenkyu-kai teachings onto her Spiritualist Church teachings to create yet another religion.[1] There was no concept of "distance" in Usui's teachings mentioned by ANY of my teachers (Mochizuki suggested that the idea had come to Japan from Reverend Takata via Mieko Mitsui).

The symbols **may well be** a state of being but they were presented to me as aspects of self connection.[2]

The point about Usui teaching no concept of distance makes perfect sense; in fact, he was teaching just the opposite—Oneness, the absence of all distance.

More from Dave King:

Historically, the association of SUN/MOON/EARTH developed as Buddhism blended with Chinese beliefs and later with folk Shinto.

Amitabha—known in Japan as Amida—is the Buddha of Infinite Light who vowed whilst still a mortal to create a pure land for other aspirants to enlightenment. The light aspect permitted Amida to be associated with Amaterasu—the Shinto Sun Goddess.

Sthamaprapta—known in Japan as Seishi—is the right hand attendant of Amida Buddha. He joins the other attendant, Kanzeon, when Amida greets newcomers to his western paradise. Seishi bestows the strength of wisdom to his devotees enabling them to break their bonds. The strength aspect was seen as a connection to Earth and its various kami (spirits).

Kanzeon (Kannon) is associated with compassion, with women and the Moon.[3]

Hiroshi Doi's Version

I don't know what Mr. Doi and the Gakkai believe about the origin of the Usui symbols, but they and others have attributed the following correlations to them:

■ **Table 7.3**

Okuden symbols and common correlations

Reiki Symbol	Celestial Body	Element	Property
#1/Focus	Earth	Earth	Physical healing
#2/Harmony	Moon	Water	Mental/emotional healing
#3/Connection	Sun	Fire	Connection: timeless/spaceless

Notice that both versions relate the symbols to Earth, Moon, and Sun, but the symbol associated with Sun in one version is associated with Moon in the other. How can this be?

William Rand tries to link the Reiki symbols to a group of three symbols used by the Kurama-Kokyo Buddhist sect (which currently maintains a temple on Mount Kurama).[4] This is a tempting correlation, because one of the Kurama symbols looks something like the Harmony symbol (Sei He Ki). Also, according to Rand, the Usui Master symbol is used by the Kurama sect to represent the Trinity of all three symbols together, which they call Sonten, the Supreme Deity and source of all creation, the spirit of the Universe. Dave King says that Rand has misunderstood this, however. He says the same kanji as the Usui Master symbol do appear in the Kurama prayer—but with a different meaning.[5] In any case, *the Kurama-Kokyo sect was not in existence until 1949, long after Usui's time.* (Mr. Rand disregards this, even though he mentions it himself.)

Looking at the Kurama symbols, we see that the one resembling Sei He Ki is called the Love symbol and represents Senju-Kannon, a Bodhisattva of Compassion. The other two are: the Power symbol, representing Mao-Son, the spirit of the Earth; and the Light symbol, representing Bishamon-ten, the spirit of the Sun. This leaves the Moon to correspond with the symbol resembling Sei He Ki.

Could these Kurama symbols be responsible for the modern-day associations attributed to the Reiki symbols by the Gakkai and others, even though it's chronologically impossible that they were the inspiration for Usui? We know the Gakkai was prohibited from meeting openly for a time, by the American military, after World War II. Taggart King says it "only reformed many years later, then consisting largely of second generation Masters, and it may be that some of the earlier teachings and practices were lost."[6]

It's quite possible that the Kurama-Kokyo Buddhists could have influenced the post-War Gakkai. The Kurama-Kokyo sect began in 1949 in a temple on Mount Kurama that was formerly maintained by the Tendai sect. Could it be that some of those second-generation Reiki

Masters, when they reformed the Gakkai, made a pilgrimage to Mount Kurama, the supposed place of Usui's Reiki awakening? If so, they would have found there, in the temple that had previously been Tendai (the sect to which Usui belonged), the following symbols:

Power: associated with Mao-son, who came to Earth from Venus six million years ago, incarnating in a cedar tree atop Kurama as the spirit of the Earth.

Love: associated with Senju-Kannon, the Bodhisattva of Compassion and Mercy, the spirit of the Moon, whose love flows out to all beings like water.

Light: associated with Bishamon-ten, the spirit of the Sun, embodiment of fire.

The Love symbol is the one that resembles Sei He Ki. It seems likely to me that this is the origin of the modern Reiki perception of Sei He Ki as Moon/Water energy; and, once that association is made, Hon Sha Ze Sho Nen becomes Sun/Fire.

What to make of all this? I offer it as the most accurate picture I've been able to piece together as to where these particular aspects of Usui's method originated and how they have come to be what they are at present.

Does it matter whether we conceptualize them as energies or states of consciousness or aspects of self-connection? Does it matter whether we associate them with Earth, Moon, and Sun and, if so, in what order? In a sheerly practical sense, it may not. The fact is, we can use these aspects of Reiki with any or none of the above perceptions and attain positive results. When I was initiated into the second level of Reiki (1991), I was taught the names of the three symbols, how to draw them and how to use them, and nothing more about them. And they worked!

I was taught to use one of them to "send distant healing"—and it worked! (Actually, I had been "sending distant healing" since my first-level initiation, because someone had tipped me off that it could be done without any symbols, merely by giving Reiki to a photo of the desired recipient.)

It seems to me, though, the more deeply we understand something, the more effectively we are able to use it. I believe that's the course of our Self-unfolding—it's a journey of ever-increasing consciousness. When I believed that I was "sending distant healing," that did appear to be what was happening. Now I believe it's more accurately a matter of realizing (as deeply as I can, with every wave-particle of my being) the existing Oneness of everything. And the effectiveness of my Reiki has increased with this realization.

I believe it's worth noticing that these three symbols—Focus, Harmony, and Oneness (I'd rather use that term than "Connection," which presupposes separation, because I believe that separation is a secondary appearance, the primary reality being Oneness)—are derived from symbols of Light, Love, and Power, whether we take the Amida Sanzon interpretation or the Kurama Sonten. Different deities are involved in either case (except Kannon, who is in both); however, the deities are merely personifications of Divine qualities. The qualities are "the deep inside"—and the qualities are the same in both cases! The personification (deity) is one step removed, and the association with Earth, Moon, or Sun is one step further removed. Understanding this, we are now able to see the wisdom of Dave King's teachers in presenting these as aspects of Self.

Does it matter then, which one—Light or Love—we associate with Sei He Ki, and which one with Hon Sha Ze Sho Nen? It matters only to the extent that one association feels more true to you than the other.

The deeper truth is that you already embody all three qualities your-self; the symbols are just "training wheels" for your awareness of that. I've used the symbols with both sets of associations—at different times, and each for a long time—with great results either way. Again, as with everything in Reiki (and in life), the crucial element is doing what feels most right in the depths of our being. We're on a path of self-discovery, of learning to be true to our Self and our Source.

Though most of Usui's students learned these aspects using koto-dama or Buddhist meditations, it seems appropriate that the method of using symbols came to the West (via Hayashi and Takata), where Shintoism and Buddhism were foreign. In the West, Reiki students have been taught to draw or envision the symbols while saying the name of the particular symbol three or four times. This indicates a recognition of the power of sound; and Mr. Doi and others even refer to the names of the symbols as their kotodama—though the names are not in fact the kotodama but were derived from them.

One of the great things about Reiki is that it encourages personal freedom. The Reiki energy itself is our greatest teacher, as it connects us increasingly with our own true, inner knowledge. The other side of this coin is the lack of standardization, which may sometimes lead to confusion. The Reiki symbols and kotodama are a good example: Hawayo Takata did not allow her students to keep written copies of the symbols; they had to rely solely on memory. As a result, different versions of the symbols appeared over time. Many of these have now been published in books, and it's remarkable how much they differ from each other. Nevertheless, they are all reported to be effective. There are even stories of people making up symbols at random, using them in place of the Reiki symbols—as an experiment—and getting comparable results.

Maybe this tells us something about the nature of symbols in general. Any particular symbol will create a characteristic vibration—but it may be that its effect has more to do with our own belief in the symbol, or the mere fact that a symbol is "shorthand" for embodying and activating our intent. In any case, I believe the most important thing is to use whatever feels most right to us; and that may change over time. Learn to trust your inner guidance—Reiki is connecting you to the Source of that.

In the Okuden initiation, we're "attuned" or "empowered" with the three aspects presented above. (Maybe it's more accurate to say that our *awareness* of these aspects—which have been within us all the time—is awakened.) Since being given the kotodama, I now give them to my students along with the symbols. I give the symbols as drawn by Hayashi-sensei. These were in the possession of Mr. Tatsumi, who allowed Dave King to trace them; and Dave has made them available to the rest of us. Please don't hesitate, though, to experiment with other versions of the symbols and compare feelings and effects. We are not attuned to particular symbols, but to what they represent. Please remember this! Don't mistake the map for the territory!

Some people say the Reiki symbols are sacred and secret, and attribute great power to them. This attitude seems to be an outgrowth of the Reiki legend, propagated in the West from the time of Takata-sensei, which described the symbols as being divinely revealed to Mikao Usui on Mount Kurama, in great, mystical balls of light. We now know that, in fact, Usui did not even introduce the symbols into his method until very near the end of his life, as aids for certain students. According to Dave King, the symbols were borrowed straight from Chinese Buddhism. ("All 4 symbols were taken to Japan from China around 600 AD and retain their original attributes. In other words Usui used the symbols in the manner used by the Chinese Buddhists."[7])

The symbols represent specific aspects and serve as focal points of our attention—a way to put the conscious mind on target. It's worth noting that, in the Usui Reiki Society in Japan, the symbols are regarded as "training wheels" on a bicycle: helpful in learning to ride, and eventually no longer needed. The kotodama can be regarded in the same way. (One of my Reiki friends, in Denmark, insists that the symbols are *sacred* training wheels!)

Drawing the Symbols

Great thanks to Dave King for providing these images, and for correcting me on the number of strokes in some of them! These were made from Dave's tracings of the symbols as presented by his teacher Tatsumi (who had them as written by Dr. Hayashi).

Cho Ku Rei

#1. Focus

(H)O (K)U E I

Grounding
Strengthening
Physical
Passive

Power
Seishi
Earth

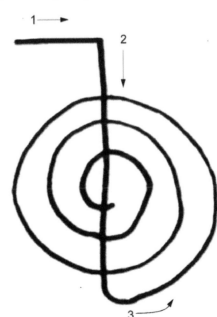

Sei He Ki

#2. Harmony

E I E I KI

Uplifting
Etheric
Psychic
Mental
Active
Heavenly

Light
Amida
Sun

Hon Sha Ze Sho Nen

#3. Connection

(H)O A ZE (H)O NE

State of consciousness: Oneness

Love

Kannon

Moon

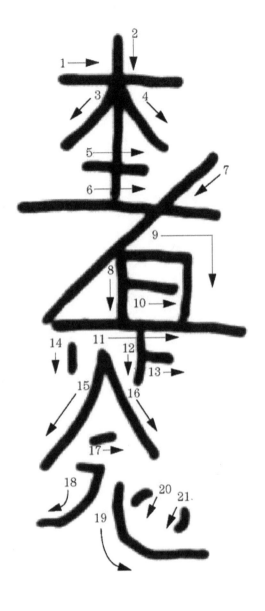

Reiki Kotodama

Until the very end of the twentieth century, only a group of students who learned from Usui-sensei directly knew about the Usui kotodama, and these former students were never affiliated with the Usui Reiki Ryoho Gakkai. Now, through those students, the world has begun to receive information on Usui's use of kotodama. And, as with the symbols, multiple versions of Usui kotodama are now circulating.[8]

Here are the Usui kotodama as learned by a student of Andy Bowling:[9]

Reiki Symbol	Kotodama
Cho Ku Rei	O U E I
Sei He Ki	E I E I KI
Hon Sha Ze Sho Nen	O A ZE O NE

The other versions I've seen are based on the same sounds, but with the addition of a few consonants. I've seen O U E I becoming HO KU E I (or HO KU EI), and O A ZE O NE becoming HO A ZE HO NE (no change to E I E I KI).

In what I've learned about kototama as taught by Nakazono-sensei, the sounds always begin as pure, individual vowel sounds and progress through a series of consonants-plus-the-vowel.[10] Nakazono presented an extensive series of sounds, comprising in its entirety a complete "Kototama Principle"—infinitely more complex than the few, individual sounds that make up the Usui kotodama. Clearly, Usui's understanding of kotodama and Nakazono's understanding of kototama seem to have been different.

Nakazono said the kototama system he learned was in use more than ten thousand years ago; and the Usui kotodama are said to come from Shinto, which originated much later. (Nakazono spelled the word as "kototama" in English, whereas the prevalent spelling, in the Reiki world, for Usui's sounds, is "kotodama.")

You might like to experiment with these different versions. Practice with each for a long enough time to feel the nature of the sounds and the effects they have on your awareness. Then you can choose what works best for you. The version with fewer consonants feels more primal, "deeper," and more effective to me. You can use symbols, kotodama, both, or neither. Just remember, they are all merely tools to shift your awareness in a particular way. The awareness is the goal; if you can achieve it directly, so much the better.

Kotodama Pronunciation

O—rhymes with "go"
U—rhymes with "blue"
E—rhymes with "day"
I—rhymes with "be"
A—rhymes with "saw"

Some people teach the sound of E as being more like the E in "well." As I practiced the kotodama, I found myself naturally drawn to using that sound, in fact. But the sound I was first taught for E was the sound of long-A (as in "day"). And the long-A sound is also what was taught by Nakazono (he described it as the sound of A in "way").

How to Make the Sounds

Here is Nakazono's description of (and reasons for) making the sounds in a particular way:[11]

> To make sounds is an action of expansion. It should start from the point of final concentration, the absolute center. That is why all Kana sounds always start with the teeth held firmly together.[12]
>
> The rhythm of sounds, our life's manifestation, is based on *I* dimension, the life will. When making the *I* sounds, the teeth remain closed; they are always made by biting the teeth.
>
> *A-O-U-E,* the four dimensions of mother sounds, and the child sounds, come out from *I*. With each sound, always return to biting the teeth.
>
> *A* sound is energy expanding to the fullest and made with a fully opened mouth. *O* sound is made with a round mouth, half closed; the smallest opening comes out as *U* sound. *I* and *E* sounds are made with the mouth open sideways. The teeth open for *E* but remain closed for *I*.

Table 7.4 incorporates kotodama, Taoist associations, Amida Sanzon associations, and Reiki symbols. The kotodama as I first learned them are in bold, with the added consonants in parentheses.

I love the simplicity of all this! In its most basic form, it's just Rei and Ki, Heaven and Earth, Great Yang and Great Yin. We could also say, Wave and Particle. And the key to the whole thing is realizing the Oneness in what appears to be duality.

Sit and focus your mind on the aspect of Earth. Get the feeling of it as much as you can. Then tone the kotodama for it. Shape your mouth to make the tones (as described above) and create the sound from the tanden by gradually tightening the hara, pushing the sound up and out. Let it happen naturally, with as little effort as possible.

■ **Table 7.4**

Okuden symbols, kotodama, Taoist and Amida Sanzon correlations

Kotodama	Taoist	Amida Sanzon	Reiki Symbol
	EARTH energy	Power	Focus
(H)O	—Heavy, grounding	deity: Seishi	
(K)U	—Strengthening body and mind	Earth	Cho
			Ku
E	—Physical healing		Rei
I	—color: Forest green		
	—Passive (Great Yin)		
	HEAVEN energy		
E	—Light, etheric	Light	Harmony
I	—Intuition	deity: Amida	
E	—Psychic awareness	Sun	Sei
I	—Mental focus		He
KI	—color: Golden		Ki
	—Active (Great Yang)		
(H)O	ONENESS	Love	Connection
A	a state of consciousness	deity: Kannon	
ZE		Moon	Hon
(H)O			Sha
NE			Ze
			Sho
			Nen

Sound each syllable equally, in monotone, as low a note as is comfortable. Let the sound resonate throughout the body. Keep toning it until you feel you have become the embodiment of Earth (or until you've had enough toning for one time!). Be fully present in the toning, and allow the process to take as long as it takes.

It was common for students of Usui to practice this every day, working with a single kotodama for months—first Earth, then Heaven, then Oneness. Please have fun with the kotodama—you can chant yourself to sleep with them, you can take them for a walk (one syllable with every step). You can experiment with enunciating every vowel sharply, and with letting them flow together slightly. You can even do them silently, in your mind. As always, let your feelings lead you; follow what feels good.

Between kotodama and symbols, there may be a fundamental difference worth noting: Kotodama are primal, Universal, pre-human sounds; written symbols came later, created by humans, therefore they are farther removed from the point of creation. Symbols *represent* things; kotodama *call things into being*. Still, remember that even the Reiki kotodama are merely "training wheels," to be used until we gain awareness directly.

Using Kotodama and/or Symbols

The realization of Oneness is the main thing to be gained from Okuden. Because of this Oneness, as we heal ourselves we are healing others inevitably. Likewise, as we heal others we are healing ourselves. All forms of life are indeed One, and we can increase our realization of this by conscious use of the Reiki kotodama and symbols.

(H)O A ZE (H)O NE and/or the "Connection" symbol can help us realize Oneness with another individual, to maximize the healing effects of Reiki, whether giving hands-on or distant treatment. It makes sense to connect with this awareness at the start of any treatment, and to remind ourselves of it during the treatment if necessary. We can do this by toning the kotodama, either aloud or mentally; by drawing the symbol in the air; by envisioning the symbol (or maybe hundreds of copies of it, filling our body or the whole room). Be creative! Let your intuition guide you!

It's interesting to note that this kotodama and symbol were associated with the Amida Sanzon symbol of Love. And what is Love but the achievement of Oneness with another being?

E I E I KI and/or the "Harmony" symbol can be especially helpful in the healing of mental/emotional aspects. I was taught to draw or envision the symbol on the back of the head while giving Reiki there. Sei He Ki has been translated by some people as "Man and God becoming One"—and Usui's initial correlation here (Taoist) was with Heaven. Also, I can't help noticing that the initial zig-zag-zig of the first stroke of the symbol makes a lightning bolt: a streak of fire, perhaps, connecting Heaven and Earth?

This kotodama and symbol were associated with the Amida Sanzon symbol of Light. Obvious correlations include enlightenment and anything dealing with the realm of consciousness, awareness, thought, and perception.

(H)O (K)U E I and/or the "Focus" symbol can help us direct energy to physical things. As the name says, the effect is to focus or concentrate energy in a single point. The symbol depicts the action of gathering energy (horizontal stroke), bringing it down (vertical stroke), and spiraling it inward to a focal point.

Numerous people have pointed out that by superimposing the symbol on the human body—with the vertical stroke along the spine, the crown chakra at the top of the spiral and the root chakra at the bottom of it—we can imagine the spiral, where it crosses the spine, passing through the seven chakras in the following order: Root, Crown, Sacral, Brow, Solar Plexus, Throat, and coming to rest at the Heart.

I was taught to draw this symbol with the spiral going in horizontal planes—and that is the way it has always felt the most "right" to me. If drawing it with the palm of the hand, for instance, the palm is held *horizontally* throughout, facing down. The horizontal stroke (#1) is made, then the vertical stroke (#2), and then the palm (still horizontal) comes up and outward from the vertical stroke of the symbol. It rises the distance of two-thirds of the vertical stroke. At this level, the spiral begins. It starts horizontally and moves downward and inward, so that—at the end of three revolutions—it finishes at the center, at a point one-third of the way up from the bottom of stroke #2.

This kotodama and symbol were associated with the Amida Sanzon symbol of Power. Obviously, when energy is concentrated or focused in a single point, power is created.

Some people in Reiki also call this the "Power" symbol, and some teach that using it in combination with the other symbols will increase their power. This may be true—though I'm not sure it's accurate to say that the symbols have power in the first place. In any case, this is not a concept that seems to have come from Usui, who used the kotodama or symbols individually.

Some people have also developed complex sequences of the symbols, sandwiching them in various ways, claiming thereby to produce many different healing effects. Again, the best advice is to follow your own intuition; if something works for you, do it!

Other Effects

I've had remarkable experiences with Hon Sha Ze Sho Nen—both in "sending" Reiki to the past and, in the present, merely by mentally projecting the symbol onto people who were set to be hostile (and suddenly became very friendly).

Other popular uses for the symbols include clearing spaces of "negative" energy, including insect pests and spirit entities (I'm told that Sei He Ki alone works amazingly well for the latter, understandably, being associated with Heaven and Light); harmonizing the energy of food before eating it (though I tend to do mine after eating, with hands on the belly); empowering beverages before drinking; clearing the road ahead when driving. In short, anything imaginable. Be creative!

Practicing the use of the kotodama and symbols can help us learn "the deep inside" of Reiki. The goal is to embody *Rei-ki*, to embody the unification of Universal Spirit and personal energy; to realize, in fact, that we have always been that unification. We can practice with the kotodama and/or symbols—and we may find that, just when we feel ready to discard them, a whole new level of understanding begins to open up. In any case, please remember, they're tools to be used only as long as they're helpful. We can use them intuitively and freshly and consciously.

The Legacy of the Symbols

There seems to be a lot of controversy and confusion about the Reiki symbols. For a long time, they were kept secret from everyone not initiated to the second level of Reiki. For decades, Reiki teachers (following in the footsteps of Hawayo Takata) did not allow their students to keep written copies of the symbols! This led to many changes in the symbols over time, from people not remembering them precisely; the imprecision was passed from teacher to student, and compounded by each generation.

Complicating things even further, Usui Reiki began to mutate into other varieties. New versions of Reiki were developed and, building on what they thought was the original model, the creators of these new varieties added more and more symbols.

At some point, a certain Reiki teacher blew the lid off the secrecy issue, by publishing a book that exposed the Reiki symbols (many variations of them) for all to see! That, in itself, created plenty of controversy. The Reiki world polarized into those who applauded the exposure, and those who thought it was sacrilege.

What no one (outside a small number of people in Japan) knew at that time was *that the Reiki symbols were not essential, or even necessary, in the first place!* And that they were not even introduced into the practice of Reiki by Mikao Usui until very near the end of his life.

Now, thanks to the work of many people giving us the ability to view a bigger picture of Usui Reiki than before, we can see how the symbols came to be used in ways that Mikao Usui had never used them, and how they came to be regarded with such mistaken importance.

Usui's final students were quite different than the others. They were military officers, possibly not accustomed to using Buddhist meditations or Shinto kotodama. And they were looking for a method of treating sickness and injuries, a method that could be learned fairly quickly by common people. So they were given symbols—to expedite and facilitate their learning. The symbols were *not* used in the Reiju empowerment procedure.

As mentioned before, Dr. Hayashi became the visible standard-bearer of Reiki after Usui's passing. In time he developed his own Reiki method, including his own initiation ceremony. His fellow students Ushida and Taketomi became, respectively, the first and second Presidents of the Usui Reiki Ryoho Gakkai. Thus, the Reiki symbols were given an importance and a function they had not had for Mikao Usui.

Years later, a Japanese-American named Hawayo Takata would become Hayashi's most famous student. She would take the role of standard-bearer after Hayashi's passing—and she would pass on his method of Reiki initiation (with modifications of her own, and calling it Attunement). This initiation ceremony featured the implanting of those famous Reiki symbols into the student's energy field! Through Takata and her lineage, this Attunement procedure of Reiki initiation has been the standard, worldwide, since the 1970s. Many variations have been born, and yet the central element of almost all seems to remain the implantation of the Reiki symbols.

All this was brought to mind one day when I received a Kundalini initiation. The giver of the initiation asked if I would like to have the Reiki symbols removed from my energy field. Her feeling was that the symbols often become obstacles to spiritual growth. On giving it some thought, and knowing that the symbols were not necessary (they were put there during Attunements I received), I couldn't see any reason to keep them. I had them removed.

This brought up other questions. Was it true that the presence of Reiki symbols in the aura could impede one's spiritual growth? Was it necessary for people to have them removed? My intuition said No— that the symbols were only symbols, and what mattered was our attitude toward them. If we viewed them as "training wheels" on a bicycle, and if we let go of them once they had served their purpose, they would not cause a problem. They would be no more than artifacts of our journey (as they were intended to be in the first place).

Of course, had the simple elegance of the Reiju empowerment merely been retained, instead of replaced by more complicated procedures (and the implanting of symbols), these artifacts would not even be there for us to contemplate; and had the Reiki symbols not been imbued with a mistaken sense of power and magic and secrecy, they would be much easier for people to let go. In fact, had Hawayo Takata found her way to another one of Usui's students than Dr. Hayashi, the world at large would not even have learned of Reiki symbols!

The moral of the story, then: Reiki symbols were intended only to be "fingers pointing at the Moon" (and the Sun, and the Earth). Let's not mistake the finger for what it's pointing at! Reiki symbols are not Reiki. It's much better to get beyond the symbols, to the Source.

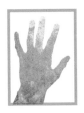

Chapter 8

More Techniques, and Usui Contemporaries

Distant Treatment

Reiki can be directed to any being, any location, any situation, any time (past, present, future). It's commonly said that we are "sending" distant healing—but I believe, more accurately, that we are "becoming" the other person, place, or situation; we are helping them to vibrate in unison with the greater Universe; we are realizing our Oneness.

We can use the "Connection" kotodama and/or symbol to help us realize our timeless, spaceless unity with the desired recipient or target. Then we simply let the Reiki flow. As in a hands-on treatment, we can either make conscious use of the other kotodama/symbols (for physical and mental/emotional healing) or not.

According to Arjava Petter, Usui-sensei taught people to use a photograph of the recipient, telling them simply to hold the photo between the palms while transmitting Reiki. Whether indeed this came from Usui or not, it does work. As already mentioned, this was the first way I learned of "sending" Reiki, before I was given the symbols. I don't know how much of its effectiveness can be attributed to the photo itself, and how much to the simple intent of the "sender." A drawing, a stick-figure, or anything else can be used as well, in place of the photo.

There are as many other methods as it's possible to imagine. Here are some popular ones:

- Use a doll or stuffed animal as a proxy for the recipient.
- Hold your hands together (with palms either touching or not quite) and imagine the recipient miniaturized between them.
- Imagine the recipient, full-size, either sitting or lying down, and perform a full treatment on this image.
- Represent the recipient with a stone or crystal or other small object—or make a representation of them (like a Native American prayer stick, for instance)—and hold it between the palms while transmitting Reiki.
- Write the recipient's name, location, age or date of birth, affirmations for healing and well-being, Reiki symbols/kotodama—any or all of these things—on a piece of paper, and hold it between the palms while transmitting Reiki.
- You can combine the previous two methods into one even more powerful by creating a "crystal grid": Choose a crystal to represent each recipient, lay them out in a meaningful pattern (such as a spiral or a geometric shape), each on top of a slip of paper with a name, location, affirmation, and Reiki symbols/kotodama. Then give the crystals Reiki for a short time every day (using kotodama and/or symbols on them, if you like). The energy will accumulate; crystals can store energy for a long time, and also concentrate it.

Again, the possible methods are limited only by your imagination. The important thing, it seems to me, is really feeling the Oneness. Do whatever gives you the strongest, most tangible feeling of the recipient, the greatest presence. Make it real.

To me, it seems natural to use my body as a proxy. I place my hands on it, with the realization that, for the purpose and duration of the Reiki session, I am One with the desired recipient.

I believe it's important, for healing in-person or at a distance, that we visualize and affirm the recipient in perfect, radiant well-being. We very likely don't even know what "perfect, radiant well-being" entails for each individual; the point is that we hold the feeling of them manifesting their perfection, whatever it happens to look like.

We must realize our true identity; that we are all Perfect, Infinite Spirit; that any kind of dis-ease or imperfection is simply not in our nature. It's impossible for Spirit to be sick or imperfect in any way! Isn't this what Mikao Usui was getting at, with his "method to achieve personal perfection"? He was looking for a way of manifesting, in this *a posteriori* world, the absolute perfection that each of us was conceived with, in the *a priori* world of Spirit! That's what Reiki—our "highest ki"—is helping us to do. *Rei-ki:* the *unification* of Universal Spirit and individual human manifestation.

This is what the greatest healers and sages have always known: that any true healing—regardless of technique or method involved—is just a matter of bringing the perfection of Spirit into the manifest world, aligning the two, realizing their Oneness. The greatest healers have seen that the *appearance* of disease is nothing more than that—in fact, a *false* appearance! And, what other people have called magic or miracles has always been merely the re-establishment of the original, true image as conceived in Spirit. Our human way of thinking is what creates our diseases. Our habitual thoughts and feelings and beliefs create our energetic vibration; and that vibration is what manifests as health or disease, abundance or lack, peace or torment. Mikao Usui knew this, when he wrote his Concepts on that piece of paper, in 1921.

It's important to remember that the removal of symptoms is not necessarily the path to well-being and is not our goal (except, possibly, in extreme crisis situations). Also, if our consciousness is focused on a symptom in any way, the effect will be to strengthen and perpetuate the symptom, not to "cure" it.

In any case, the Reiki will flow and the natural intelligence of the recipient's body will direct it for the maximum benefit. I don't believe our thoughts and feelings alter significantly the working of Reiki, but they have very powerful effects of their own, which work either with the Reiki or against it. If we're giving someone Reiki, though picturing them as being ill, our thoughts of illness are actually countering the healing effects of the Reiki. By the same token, the person's own thoughts and self-image are even more powerful and pervasive. As long as a person pictures himself habitually as being unwell, or dwells in any sort of negative, low-vibrational thinking—involving fear, anger, worry, confusion, criticism, depression, sadness, and such—no amount or kind of "treatment" from anyone will be able to heal him. (I've learned, much better than I ever wanted to, the total devastation that results when we let ourselves be sucked into the whirlpool of emotional traumas for a long enough time. Been there, done that, got the T-shirt to prove it!)

Distant treatments are usually given for shorter periods of time than hands-on—often much shorter, as little as a few minutes. This may be because a stronger mental focus is required with the recipient not physically present. Still, I find it not difficult to hold the focus for times approaching those of hands-on treatments. I believe it's good practice, in fact. Also, the distance doesn't have to be a long one: You can treat someone sitting a few feet away from you. It's even been said that Usui had a special fondness for distant treatment and would often treat someone from an adjacent room.

Asking Permission

Some people are very strict about not "sending" distant Reiki unless the recipient has given them permission. I believe this is generally a wise policy. As with other kinds of help, it seems best that we let people know it's available and then allow them to request it. There are times, though—when we become aware of sudden injuries or emergencies, for instance—that obtaining permission is not feasible, and yet we feel strongly drawn to offer Reiki. Similarly, we may feel drawn to offer it to regions of the Earth, to nations and the leaders of nations, etc.—where it's not feasible to ask permission personally. In these cases, I believe it's quite all right to offer Reiki. It is indeed an offering; I don't believe Reiki can ever be forced on beings against their will. Anyone who doesn't at some level desire it will simply not receive it.

Arjava Petter told a story about feeling that he was receiving some kind of oppressive energy at one point in his life, before he became interested in Reiki. He was in India at the time. He later learned that his brother in Germany had been secretly "sending" him Reiki—and Arjava believed that was causing his feeling of oppression. My own inclination is that it was not the Reiki but perhaps the willful intent of his brother's thoughts. The brother wanted Arjava to learn Reiki and was trying to push him in that direction.

I believe it's important to distinguish here what is Reiki and what isn't. Reiki is a very high-level, intelligent, and loving energy, which I believe will never in any case be an instrument of harm or oppression.

Our personal egos, on the other hand, are generally functioning with less intelligence (though we may not like to admit it) and their own selfish agenda. We very often slip into the habit of trying to control people and events; and our personal will can be strong enough to do this, to some extent. I believe the application of our will to bring about certain results is what actually causes problems and creates the feeling of negative or oppressive energy in a recipient. It's of utmost importance that we monitor ourselves in this regard, to ensure that our thoughts (which are enormously powerful) work to enhance the effects of the Reiki, not to counteract them. It's important that we not try to bring about a preconceived result.

Usui Stone Method

Here's a healing technique using stones, which Taggart King says was utilized by Usui-sensei. The following stones are used:

- Clear Quartz: empowered with the Connection kotodama and placed on the Brow Chakra
- Citrine: empowered with the Focus kotodama and placed on the Throat Chakra
- Jade (preferably unpolished): empowered with the Harmony kotodama and placed on the Heart Chakra

Each stone can be empowered by holding it, toning the kotodama three times, and letting the energy flow for as long as you like. Of course, you can tone the kotodama continuously if you prefer. I like to cup the stone in both hands and bring them up to the mouth, so I'm toning the kotodama right into the stone. Then I breathe Reiki into it with three long, slow, *hado* breaths.

The stones are put in place and left during the treatment. My experience has been that the stones give a marvelous treatment all by themselves. I simply put them in place, remaining present myself (a few feet away), and let them work. It's helpful to refresh their empowerment before every use.

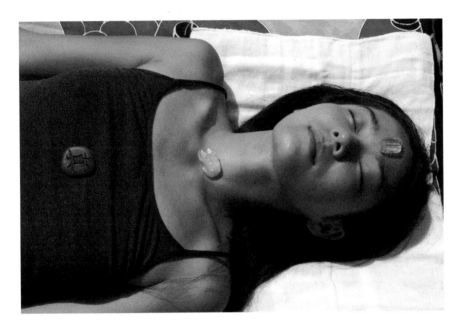

Contemplating the workings of the stones, and why they are placed as they are, led me to create the following table:

■ **Table 8.1**

Relation of Usui stones to kotodama/symbols, qualities, and chakra energies

Stone:	JADE	QUARTZ	CITRINE
Kotodama/ Symbol:	E I E I KI Harmony	(H)O A ZE (H)O NE Connection/Oneness	(H)O (K)U E I Focus
Qualities/ associations:	Light or Heaven	Love or Oneness	Power
	Sun	Moon (whose light is the reflection of the Sun)	Wisdom
	Enlightenment		Earth
	"Man and God becoming One"		Physicality

Chakra:	HEART	BROW	THROAT
Energy centered in this chakra:*	Denki/ "Thunder"	Reiki/ "Spirit"	Jiki/ "Magnetic" or "Gathering"
	which implies Heaven & allows relationship with a Divine Source	which connects us to Source and directs all energies below it	Polarity, vibration, materialization
		As Mr. Doi says, "Reiki is wave of Love!"	

* For a description of the seven energies in the body, see "*Ki*, the Energy of Life," in Chapter 5.

Usui Contemporaries

Renowned for his abilities in several martial arts, Mikao Usui was a contemporary and friend of other famous martial artists: Jigoro Kano, founder of Judo; Gichin Funakoshi, founder of modern Karate-do; and Morihei Ueshiba, founder of Aikido—to name a few.

Jigoro Kano

Jigoro Kano, the founder of Judo, was a friend and mentor of Usui. Born in 1860, just five years before Usui, he studied literature, economics, philosophy, and political science at the Emperor's University in Tokyo, later becoming a teacher and school principal. He dedicated his life to education. He founded the Tokyo Teachers' Training College and was the head of it for thirty years.

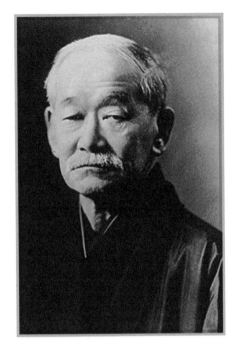

Jigoro Kano
Image courtesy www.judo1.nl/

In 1882 (the year Mokichi Okada, the founder of Johrei, was born), Kano opened his first dojo. He began teaching what he called Judo, his own integration of many other methods. More than just a martial art, Judo was designed to provide physical, mental, and moral education. It was a *Do* (a "Way" of life), based on principles of gentleness and flexibility, with the aim of total self-improvement.

According to Dave King, Usui was influenced greatly by Jigoro Kano: "Usui made use of the judojo rituals and gradings as developed by Kano." The version of Usui-do learned by Dave includes a ceremonial "rite of passage" (called Transformation) between levels. He emphasizes that this was not Reiju. He says Usui seems to have taken this rite of passage from Shinto, and that Jigoro Kano was involved in leading him to it.[1]

Omoto Kyo, the Deguchis, Mokichi Okada and Johrei

Mokichi Okada joined the Omoto Kyo religion in 1918 or 1920 (different sources give different dates). In late 1926 (about nine months after the passing of Mikao Usui) he began having spiritual revelations. A "torrent" of "words about things I could not have imagined" began to pour out of him.

This was the start of a huge transformation in Okada. He later wrote, "Some enormous power was moving me freely at its will. A step at a time I came to grasp the reality of the realm of God through various miracles." And, "The more that I doubted, the more miracles occurred to dispel my doubts."

"In my abdomen there is a sphere of light," he wrote. "This is the spirit of one of the highest of the divine beings." It made itself known as the spirit of the Bodhisattva Kannon, in fact. "Using me as its instrument," Okada wrote, "it orders me to help each and every living creature."[2] He began to help by devoting himself to the practice of *chinkon kishin*, an ancient Shinto meditation resurrected by Omoto Kyo. By repeating this practice, it was supposed that one might receive strength from divine entities to heal illness and even to perform miracles.

Okada soon discovered that he indeed had the ability to heal even so-called incurable diseases. Word spread, and he became busier and busier practicing this *chinkon* with people. In 1928 he retired from active participation in his business, Okada Enterprises. He had also begun to realize that his spiritual growth was taking him beyond the boundaries of Omoto Kyo—though he remained a member of Omoto

OMOTO KYO

Nao Deguchi and her adopted son Onisaburo (original name Kisaburo Ueda) founded a religion called Omoto Kyo. In 1892 Nao became possessed by a spiritual entity who claimed to be God (Ushitora no Konjin). Though illiterate herself, Nao began doing (when the spirit was present) automatic writings. These became the scriptures of Omoto Kyo. By the time of her death in 1918, Nao Deguchi had produced some two hundred thousand pages of automatic writing (none of which she was ever able to read)!

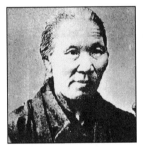 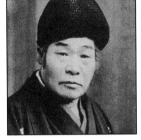

Nao Deguchi   **Onisaburo Deguchi**
Both images courtesy The Moon of Onisaburo Deguchi
(www2.plala.or.jp/wani-san/)

The possessing spirit, Ushitora no Konjin, had predicted that Nao would meet a man who would be instrumental in conveying the message of Ushitora no Konjin to the world. In 1898, at age sixty-one, she met Kisaburo Ueda (age twenty-seven)—and the spirit insisted that he was the man. On January 1, 1900, Kisaburo married Nao's daughter Sumiko. He changed his name to Onisaburo Deguchi and became the co-founder of Omoto Kyo, which is still active today.[3]

until 1934. Shortly before that, he refined his chinkon method of healing and began calling it Okada-Style Spiritual Finger-Pressure Therapy (which conjures up a very different image than the way in which Johrei is given today). The term "Johrei" was not used by Okada until much later, 1947. It's been said that Okada and Onisaburo Deguchi (one of Omoto Kyo's founders) were both students of Mikao Usui in the 1920s.

Part Three

The Mystery
(Shinpiden)

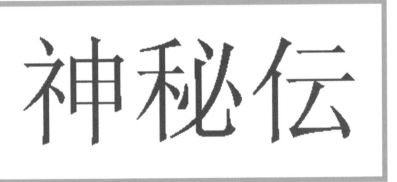

Kanji image courtesy Dave King

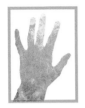

Chapter 9

Great Bright Light

Dai Ko Myo

Dai Ko Myo is the Usui "Master" symbol. It relates to Dainichi Nyorai, the Supreme Buddha, creator and Great Light of the Universe. What it really symbolizes, I believe, is our connection with the Source of All That Is—whether we call the Source Buddha, God, Allah, or anything, or nothing. At the Shinpiden (third) level, we deepen and strengthen awareness of this connection.

We have seen that the other three Reiki symbols were associated with Buddhist deities of Light, Love, and Power—individual aspects of the Supreme Buddha. The Master symbol, representing Dainichi, incorporates all these aspects. We've already come to realize these as aspects of ourselves. Each of us is a perfect and unique extension of divine Source; therefore, all the aspects of Source are present in our fundamental nature.

Shinpiden ("The Mystery") is about consolidating these aspects in ourselves and adding one more, the aspect of Empowerment. In Shinpiden, we receive the ability to perform Reiki empowerments.

We have seen that the Okuden symbols, while not *representing* the energies of Earth, Sun, and Moon, are associated with them by exten-

大
光
明

sion (by representing deities associated with them). By further extension, they also relate to the elements of Earth, Fire, and Water.

Dai Ko Myo, the kanji, depict literally, "Great Light Sun-and-Moon." Together, they are usually translated as "Great Bright Light." The implication of a Source of such Light begs our attention. From the Source comes everything, including our empowerment and, eventually, our ability to empower self and others.

By extension we have related the Okuden symbols to the elements of Earth, Fire, and Water. It's commonly taught that Dai Ko Myo, representing the Source of All That Is, incorporates all these. It seems to me there is another aspect or element as well, one which is crucial in Dai Ko Myo: the element of Air, the aspect of Breath or Soul. This aspect is more subtle (more spiritualized, less materialized) than the other three, hence more powerful. I view it as the crucial aspect involved in the ability to give empowerment (just as the Creator deity, whatever its name, is often perceived as breathing the Breath of Life into its creations).

Usui's Master Level

As taught by Mikao Usui (at least to a number of his students in Japan), the highest levels of training encompassed the following:

- receiving further spiritual teachings, by studying Buddhist sutras
- receiving regular Reiju empowerments
- receiving other, "higher" empowerments
- learning self-empowerment methods
- working with a fourth kotodama, the Empowerment kotodama
- practicing a sequence of meditations or energy exercises to further spiritual awareness and lead to *satori* (moments of sudden

understanding, insights that bring about fundamental changes of consciousness).

Eventually, near the end of Master training, the student learned how to perform Reiju and "higher empowerments."[1] In the words of Taggart King, "This may have been described as 'Shihan' level. The system was open-ended, though: you never completed it; it was a lifetime journey. It was about defining and finding your place cosmically."

He also says: "It is sometimes claimed that Usui taught Mastership at seven levels. It is a matter of interpretation really: the various meditations that you carried out totaled seven, and I suppose you could say that when you were working on meditation #2 you were at level 2, and when you reached meditation #4 you were at level 4, but this is irrelevant really."[2]

Empowerment Symbol and Kotodama

As we already know, Usui introduced symbols into his method near the very end of his life, to help certain students. The Okuden symbols were called Focus, Harmony, and Connection. The Master symbol was called Empowerment. Most of his students were given Buddhist meditations and/or Shinto kotodama instead, to help focus their awareness on these aspects of themselves. The empowerment kotodama and symbol relate to the deity Dainichi Nyorai (Mahavairocana, Great Shining One).

Taggart King says:

Dainichi Nyorai is the embodiment of Illumination (enlightenment) and represents the Universe in its ultimate form, totality and reality. Through his life force he maintains the creation and operation of the Universe and all things emerge from and are nourished by him.

And further:

The core teaching of the Mahavairocana sutra is that Enlightenment is simply "to know one's mind as it truly is." The way to achieve this, it says, is to have a mind bent towards enlightenment, to be motivated solely by compassion, and to be expedient in practice to the last.

The empowerment kotodama represented creative energy, regenerative energy, the energy of rebirth. The idea here is that when Reiju is carried out, it connects the recipient to the energy, allowing them to be "reborn": reborn in the sense of creating a place within that is "what we originally were," the state within the ovum when we were Divine essence in complete connection to the universe. The energy was the essence of earth and heavenly energy, white light, source, ultimate being.

Usui was far from unique in relating Dai Ko Myo to such ultimate being or light. Among the myriad of disciplines practiced by Usui during his lifetime was one called Shugendo ("Way of Cultivating Spiritual Powers"). Shugendo itself was a blend of many other systems, and Usui's first connection with Dai Ko Myo may have been there. One of the deities in Shugendo is Fudo Myo, one of the five Buddha aspects. Fudo Myo is the "guardian of the light," and he wears a medallion with Dai Ko Myo—the "key to the light"—on it.

The Empowerment kotodama, as I learned it (from a student of Andy Bowling), is: **A U I O.** Since then I've seen it being taught in two other ways: A I KO YO and A-I KU YO. Pronunciation is the same as with the Okuden kotodama:

A—rhymes with "saw"
U—rhymes with "blue"

I—rhymes with "be"

O—rhymes with "go"

The Empowerment symbol and kotodama both can be used, either separately or together, as tools for empowerment—first of all, within yourself, to establish your connection with Source energy. Once that is established, you can use them with empowerment procedures, such as Reiju, to help connect others.

Drawing the Symbol

Dai Ko Myo

#4. Empowerment

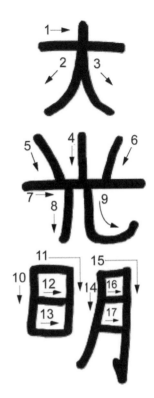

What Really Happens in a Reiki Empowerment?

Of all the Reiki mysteries, this may be the most mysterious. I certainly cannot provide the definitive answer to this question. I can only offer my personal observations and intuitions, but I feel it's a subject worth exploring.

When I received my first-level initiation, I was given four Attunements—the connotation being that my personal vibratory frequency was being "tuned" to a certain wavelength, almost like tuning a radio to a particular station. It seemed a rather magical process, and one that required obvious effort from the teacher. He took in a great breath of air and held it for the duration of the procedure, and this created a palpable sense of urgency about the whole thing: He had to do the Attunement as quickly as possible so he could breathe again!

As it happened, this was also the first Attunement method I learned myself, years later. I discovered that it was even more difficult than just holding the breath; at the same time, the anal sphincter had to be held tightly closed for the duration of the Attunement. This was in order to close an "energy gate" at the Root Chakra, called the Hui Yin.

At some point I learned that this procedure was derived from a Chi-gung exercise. When and by whom it was introduced into Reiki, I don't know (but, apparently, somewhere in the Hayashi-Takata lineage). Basically, the idea behind it was for the teacher to take in as much energy (with the breath) as possible, concentrate it in the tanden, hold it there, and seal off all the bodily exits. Then, by intent, this trapped energy (plus Reiki symbols) could be projected out through the hands, into the aura of the student, resulting in Attunement.

As we know, Mikao Usui was a Kiko Master, among other things. He spent years and years practicing numerous energy disciplines. I'm sure he was quite expert himself at doing this kind of thing. But I've seen no evidence that he made this a part of his "method to achieve personal perfection."

It seems to me that the defining characteristic of Usui's method, and its great innovation and advantage over many others, is that it gets beyond the strategy of "storing" energy. Instead, it's a method of unifying the flow of our personal energy with that of the greater Universe. Or, we might say it as: tapping into the Source of all energy, being an open conduit (a "hollow bone," as some have said) for that. So there's no need to hold our breath; in fact, that seems counterproductive. When we're "plugged in" to the Source of all energy—which is infinite and limitless and inexhaustible—the concept of accumulating or "storing" energy makes no sense!

And yet, the Attunements given to me with the Chi-gung technique were effective. I did feel different, as though my vibrational pattern had changed; I felt "at home"—in my body and in the world—more than I had before; and I was transmitting tangible energy through my palms. I truly was attuned to a different vibration than before (though I've come to wonder if it was *despite* the Chi-gung technique more than because of it!).

In subsequent years I would learn that there are many other styles of Attunement (in fact, everyone who gives Attunements probably does them a little bit differently). Apparently (no surprise!) the physical motions of the procedure are not the important part. In fact, empowerment can be given with no physical procedure at all, merely by intent.

So, then, what's the key that makes it work? Is it the Empowerment symbol, Dai Ko Myo, the Shugendo "key to the light"? No—because Usui was giving and teaching "empowerment" without the use of any symbol. But ... maybe he was using the Empowerment kotodama instead. Would it be accurate to say that one or the other, symbol or kotodama, is necessary for conveying empowerment?

I would say not. Nor are kotodama and/or symbols sufficient, in themselves, to empower anyone. Like the other symbols and kotodama, the Empowerment symbol and kotodama are merely tools to increase our awareness of attributes within ourselves.[3] We are born with a connection to limitless empowerment, we are extensions of pure, infinite Source. All that's missing is our *realization* of that. We can look at the Reiki symbols and kotodama as pointing to the buds of Harmony, Connection, Focus, and Empowerment already inside us. The more attention and reverence we give them, the wider they open—and the more aligned we become with our cosmic purpose and the power of the greater Universe.

It's important to keep in mind that each Reiki "empowerment" is an initiation to a new level of ourselves—not the end, only the beginning. Our work lies in realizing, in the most literal sense of the word, our own true nature. So, empowerment is really a continual process, not a single event. Nonetheless, it's a process enhanced by the Empowerment ceremony. How does this work?

It seems to me that our ability to give empowerment depends very much on our having developed the qualities of Harmony, Connection, and Focus that were the subjects of Okuden. I see Harmony as our link to "Heaven," Connection (Oneness or Love) as our link to other earthly beings, and Focus as the point of intersection of the two: a point in space and time, in which we consciously bring Heaven and Earth together.

Just as our ability to bring healing to another depends on our realization of Oneness, so it is (I believe) with the ability to give empowerment. First we must establish our own connection with Source, then with the person to be empowered. The Source changes our own vibration and, through us, the vibration of the other person. The Empowerment symbol and kotodama can be used as tools for helping us connect with Source, but they are not themselves the connection.

Our effectiveness in empowering others depends on how well we have aligned our own lives with Universal truth. How much fear and worry do we live with? How much anger? How much love and gratitude? Reiki "Mastery" is really mastery of ourselves. Even to aspire to this level, I feel, requires a daily commitment to living the Concepts, working consciously with the energy, and discovering and fulfilling our life's purpose. Reiki "empowerment" does not come from any sort of magic formula, any series of movements or symbols or mudras; it's a matter of attaining a state of Oneness ourselves—bringing *Rei* and *ki* together—and then conferring that energetic reality upon someone else.

Empowerment Procedures

As already stated, I feel that the Empowerment symbol works on a more subtle level than the other three: the level of Air, the "Breath of God," which breathes life into our Soul. Being the most subtle, this Breath is also the most powerful.

The physical procedure used in giving empowerment is merely a ceremonial form, a way of directing the energy. This is why there are countless variations in procedure and yet all of them can be effective. In fact, a physical procedure of any kind is not even necessary. As I see it, the crucial elements for effectiveness are:

- Love: our degree of Oneness with the other person
- Intent: that the person truly receive empowerment, a change of vibration, change of consciousness
- Humility: the acknowledgment that we are not the source of empowerment, only the conduit
- Understanding: as true a concept as possible of the nature of the Universe and ourselves, and of what we are doing in the empowerment process

The first three of these elements are self-evident. Regarding the fourth, I would like to offer some of my current thoughts—pointing out that my own understanding continues to change—and a description of an empowerment procedure based on my "You Are The Universe!" concept.

First, though, a little background on traditional empowerment.

Usui Reiju

This is the empowerment procedure that was given to the Japanese students who have been teaching Chris Marsh. According to them, it comes from Tendai Buddhism. Receiving Reiju regularly and often (for example, weekly) was a key element in their training (and very different from receiving Attunements only as one-time initiations at each level, which became the procedure with Hayashi and Takata). Receiving Reiju repeatedly serves as a frequent cleansing of our energy field, continuing to enhance our alignment with the greater Universe.

As with giving Reiki "treatment," it seems to me most helpful to practice the empowerment procedure repeatedly on ourselves before giving it to others. I recommend to my students (at Shinpiden level) that they give themselves Reiju every day, at least until they feel at home enough with it to give it to others. In addition to increasing our confidence and our intuitive understanding of the process—once again, the Reiki energy itself is our very best teacher—doing Reiju (whether for self or others) is a great way to raise one's vibration! Also, there comes the realization that, really, there are no "others." Everything we see as *other* is really a projection of some aspect of the Self.

For several years I've been doing a lot of "distant" Reiju with people all over the world. My usual way of doing it has been as self-Reiju (with the realization that myself and the "other" are One). In fact, the self-Reiju procedure has become my usual way of doing "distant" Reiki "treatment" as well. I really cannot see a distinction between "treatment" and "empowerment," as far as what is happening energetically. I still give in-person treatments in the customary, hands-on way—because people (myself included) enjoy that way—but I know the healing could just as well be brought about in other ways.

I will not describe the Reiju procedure here; that is taught individually, when people reach the Shinpiden level. For those readers who have already learned a Reiju procedure, I can offer a few suggestions for using it. For one thing, you may like to do Reiju—or even just the preliminary step—to raise your vibration and prepare the space before giving a Reiki treatment or a Western-style Attunement, or as a way of energetically purifying any space.

Also, you can use Reiju in a particular way for empowerments at each level—Shoden, Okuden, and Shinpiden—instead of Western-style Attunements.

Using Reiju at Each Level

At all levels, Reiju was given many times to some of Usui's students, regularly and often. According to the students Chris Marsh has learned from, the Shoden empowerment was done with basic Reiju and simply the intention of opening the energy path so the student could receive whatever he or she needed for maximum benefit. In addition to receiving Shoden empowerments, the student would practice meditations designed to enhance awareness of the hara.

At Okuden, there were meditations (used by the Buddhist students) to help one "become" Earth energy and Heaven energy and Oneness. The empowerment procedure might be basic Reiju again, or it could involve the use of kotodama. In that case, there would be a series of three empowerments: giving Reiju while intoning, silently, the Focus kotodama (during the first Reiju), then the Harmony kotodama (during the second Reiju), then the Connection kotodama (during the third Reiju). The kotodama could be intoned either three times each or throughout the whole Reiju procedure.

After these empowerments, if the students were followers of Shinto, they would spend time every day toning the kotodama—working with each one until they were ready for the next—to achieve the same "becoming" that other students achieved with the Buddhist meditations.

At Shinpiden level, there were similar options. Empowerment could be given through basic Reiju, with the intention that the student receive the ability to empower others; or the kotodama technique could be used, this time with the Empowerment kotodama. In either case, there were accompanying meditations or toning of kotodama by the students at this level.

My Own Variation

My own intuitive way of using Reiju at Shoden level has been to give a series of four empowerments, intoning a kotodama with each one: Focus first, then Harmony, then Connection, then Empowerment. In a way, this seems like combining Okuden and Shinpiden empowerments into one; but the student has no conscious knowledge of the kotodama or symbols or individual aspects of the energy at this point, and the intent of the empowerment is simply to open the student's connection to all aspects of the energy, to the greatest extent possible.

I like to make the connection with each aspect individually, even though the student is not consciously aware of it. My feeling is that the Focus aspect empowers the Physical body, the Harmony aspect empowers the Mental body, the Connection aspect empowers the Emotional body, and the Empowerment aspect empowers the Spiritual body. I believe intuitively that this is why Takata gave four Attunements at first level.

At Okuden level, I give three empowerments—using the Focus, Harmony, and Connection kotodama.

At Shinpiden level, I give the same four empowerments as at Shoden. The difference is, my intent is now that the student be given the ability to empower others; and the student has of course already incorporated the aspects of Focus and Harmony and Connection at a conscious level (and will now do so with the Empowerment aspect).

"Distant" Reiju

Naturally, if we can "send" Reiki treatment through space and time, we can "send" Reiki empowerment as well. There are surely countless ways of doing it. You can use a doll or a stuffed animal toy as a proxy for the recipient; you can use a picture of the recipient; you can simply visualize the recipient sitting in front of you, and perform Reiju.

Whether sending treatment or empowerment, I believe the effects of the Reiki are enhanced by the conscious cooperation of the recipient. Therefore, I ask people to name a day and time when they can be undisturbed and consciously receptive. Most of them feel the energy very strongly this way; and, even though I spend no more than ten minutes giving Reiju, people often continue perceiving energy movement for an hour or more.

Since the "sending" is really a matter of realizing the Oneness of All, it seems most natural to me to "send" empowerment via self-Reiju. I either stand, or sit in seiza. I connect consciously with Source, and give thanks for All That Is. Then I connect with (or "become") the other person before starting the preliminary step of Reiju.[4]

I see Time as merely a fourth dimension, a coordinate that can be matched with a physical location. So I begin by saying to myself: "For the purpose and duration of this Reiju, I realize total Oneness with this (person's name, location and/or other identifying attributes), for the greatest awareness, greatest empowerment, greatest Self-realization." If I know the recipient personally or have a photo, I visualize the person as I'm saying the name. Then I specify the time this is to be perceived by the recipient (including year, month, day of the week, and day of the month).

Then I perform self-Reiju as usual, focusing on the feeling of oneness with the other person. Then I thank the recipient and bless him or her. Then I thank divine Source again.

A wonderful thing about this is that I don't have to "send" at the same time the other person is receiving. If the person is halfway around the world from me and wants to receive Reiju when it's 3 a.m. my time, it's no problem; I can do my part whenever it's convenient for me. I don't even need to know the amount of time difference between us. All I need to do is set the Reiju to be perceived at the desired time. The person will perceive it then, even if I don't "send" it until later![5] Some people don't set a time at all for "sending" Reiki or Reiju, they just do their part whenever convenient and expect the recipient to do likewise. But my experience has been that the procedure is more effective (or at least perceived more clearly) when both people have agreed upon a time.

Also, as mentioned already, Reiju can be done merely by intent—in the blink of an eye, with no physical procedure at all. And I'm finding, more and more, that this kind of not-doing usually gives the best results!

We can also—as with Reiki "treatment"—send Reiju to ourselves in the past or future. We can send it to a future time when we're expecting to be especially tired or vulnerable or experiencing some kind of stress or difficulty; or to a past time when something traumatic or harmful happened to us. The most spectacularly wonderful experience I've ever had with "distant" Reiki came from sending it to a place and time sixteen years in someone's past.

"Healing" Attunements

Somewhere along the path of Reiki's evolution, someone came up with the idea of a "Healing Attunement": a procedure in the form of Attunement, but with the intent of healing, not empowerment. I suppose it seemed a good idea at the time, but looking at it now, it makes no sense to me.

According to the students teaching Chris Marsh, Usui's procedure was to give people Reiju every time they came to him for treatment. He would empower them in this way so they could give themselves Reiki from the very beginning. This is so obviously the most sensible and helpful thing to do. And, sadly, it seems the only reason it has not been done in the West (and probably not by others in Japan, either) is the desire to keep people coming back for treatments, and, if they want empowerment, to make them pay extra for it!

It seems this mentality is what produced the concept of a Healing Attunement—the idea being that it was more powerful than a normal Reiki treatment, but it would not confer the ability to give Reiki to oneself.

Beyond the stinginess of this approach, it makes no sense to me simply because any distinction between healing and empowerment is artificial, as I see it. Healing *is* empowerment, empowerment *is* healing. How can we set the two apart? I've begun giving empowerments to people when I treat them and showing them my "You Are The Universe!" self-treatment method.

The other side of the coin is that when people ask me to "send" healing, I do it in the form of Reiju—simply intending the "greatest healing, awakening, empowerment," or whatever the person has asked to receive. It seems to me there really is no distinction: Reiju is a great healing treatment as well as an empowerment.

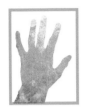

Chapter 10

Alternative Energies

Energy Concepts

Various philosophies and civilizations have conceptualized energy in different ways. The ancient Chinese Taoists developed a system of Five Transformations (literally, five "journeys"). The not-quite-so-ancient Greeks had a system of four Mundane Elements, with a Spiritual or Etheric element above them. I've not studied either of these systems deeply, but contemplating what I do know about them has led me to a system of my own.

First let's look at some old ideas, then I'll present my own modern synthesis.

The Chinese System

The five phases of energy, or Transformations, are: Water, Tree, Fire, Earth, Metal. These are seen to interact in two simultaneous cycles, a Generative (sometimes called Creative) cycle and a Controlling (sometimes called Destructive) cycle.

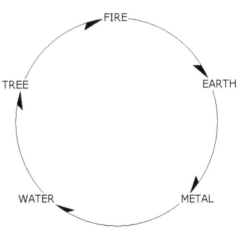

Generative cycle

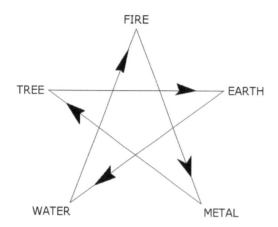

Controlling cycle

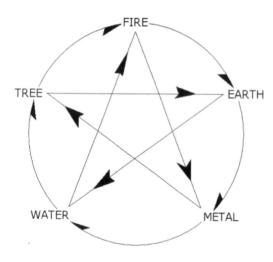

**Generative and Controlling
cycles together**

In the Generative cycle, Water generates (or is transformed into) Tree; Tree generates (or is transformed into) Fire; Fire generates (or is transformed into) Earth; Earth generates (or is transformed into) Metal; and Metal generates (or is transformed into) Water. The whole process is a circle.

In the Controlling cycle, Water controls Fire; Fire controls Metal; Metal controls Tree; Tree controls Earth; Earth controls Water. Like the Generative cycle, this is a continuous process with no beginning or end. When diagrammed, it forms a five-pointed star.

The cycles are superimposed in the diagram to the left.

The understanding is that energy is constantly changing form, "journeying" from one of these five to another, and this is how the Universe maintains balance. For example: An excess of energy in the form of Water will create new Tree energy; and, at the same time, energy in the form of Earth will exert a controlling influence on the excessive Water.

This seems logical enough, and observable in the natural environment. These energies or Transformations are also seen to take place in the human body (as well as in plants and other animals). Much of

Traditional Chinese Medicine is based on this. But it seems to me that something is missing here.

The Five Transformations form a closed system. A certain amount of intelligence is obviously present; the five forms of energy do a wonderful job of balancing each other. But they seem forever stuck in their cycle, like an ingenious, perpetual-motion machine that someone has created and set into action. They will go on transforming forever—unless the Creator steps in and dismantles them or changes the system. They will keep transforming and transforming—but with no possibility of evolving in any way.

What's missing is the connection to a Source. We're looking at the Universe as a closed container, with a finite amount of energy sealed inside, energy that merely recycles itself forever, with nowhere to go, nothing to grow into. I suppose the Taoists would disagree with me, but I see this as a rather mechanical and unrealistic view of life. To me, the fundamental element in any realistic view—the *sine qua non*—is the Source. In the Five Transformations theory, the Source is missing!

In Chapter 5 (the section called *"Ki,* the Energy of Life"), we looked at a Japanese system of seven hierarchical energies in the human body, centered in the chakras One through Six. If we apply the Five Transformations to the chakra system, where will these five forms of energy be centered?

The Root Chakra seems the natural center of Earth energy.
The Sacral Chakra seems the natural center of Water energy.
The Solar Plexus Chakra is surely the natural center of Fire energy.

What about Metal and Tree energies? In the Generative cycle, Metal is between Earth and Water—which would center it between the Root and Sacral chakras in the body. In the Generative cycle, Tree is between Water and Fire—which would center it between the Sacral and Solar Plexus chakras in the body.

Alternatively, looking at the Controlling cycle, Metal is between Fire and Tree—putting it still somewhere in the abdomen; and Tree is between Metal and Earth—putting it even lower in the abdomen.

With either cycle, then, we have all five energies within the realm of the first three chakras. This does seem quite fitting: The first three chakras involve the fundamentals of physical existence and relationship, which is exactly what the Five Transformations are all about. The awareness of more subtle, spiritual aspects of life, and of a spiritual Source of everything, and of our connection with that Source, does not arise until the opening of the fourth chakra, the Heart! And at that point, it seems we need to introduce additional elements, in order to have an accurate understanding.

What about the Greeks?

The Greeks also described a system of five elements, though not quite the same ones. They had four "mundane" elements—Earth, Water, Air, and Fire—and an additional, more subtle element—Spirit or Ether. I'm not aware of a Generative cycle or a Controlling cycle among these elements, only that they were described in terms of their subtlety and the properties of heat, cold, dryness, and wetness, and of relationships to seasons of the year. There was indeed a concept of Spirit, but it's not clear that the organizers of this system really knew what to do with it. It was described in one piece I read as a "nebulous nothingness" that was considered to be located somewhere "above" the four mundane elements, and considered not to have any bearing on human health!

My intuitive understanding of Universal elements and their corre-
lation with the human microcosm (see "You Are The Universe!" in
Chapter 3) involves these same four mundane elements, though the
Greeks ranked them slightly differently in terms of subtlety. From most
subtle to most material, they list the elements as: Fire, Air, Water, Earth.
It seems to me that Air is the most subtle, followed by Fire, Water, and
Earth. A look at the human body appears to confirm this:

Earth energy, obviously the most dense, is centered in the Root
Chakra; Water energy, slightly less dense, is centered in the Sacral
Chakra; the next chakra is the Solar Plexus, obviously the home of Fire
energy; and the next is the Heart Chakra, responsible for the heart and
lungs, which are powered by Air and Breath.

Also, it seems apparent by simply observing fire itself that Fire is
more substantial and cohesive than Air.

My Own System

It's my nature to be eclectic, and it seems to me that we can get a more
accurate understanding of reality than either the Chinese or Greek system by combining parts of both. For starters, I see that both contain
Earth and Water and Fire energies, which are clearly associated with
the first three chakras—just as in my perception of "You Are The Universe!" Then the Greek system includes Air—another of my "Universe"
elements—which can be paired appropriately with the fourth chakra.
This leaves Metal and Tree and Spirit/Ether to consider:

The step from Water to Fire has always seemed a big one to me, and
Tree (as in the Chinese system) is the perfect bridge between the two.
So now I have Earth, Water, Tree, Fire, and Air.[1] What about Spirit/Ether?

I would say Spirit is the most essential and powerful element of all;
that nothing can exist physically without first existing spiritually. And

I would say that Spirit is definitely not a "nebulous nothingness." And it is the *primary* element in human health. But where to center it in the body? And what exactly is meant by "Ether"?

I believe this Ether is right on the borderline between physical and spiritual, if such a thing is possible. Clearly it is more subtle than Air and would be centered above Air in the body. How convenient that the very next chakra, the Throat, is the center of Magnetism and Vibration!—which I would call qualities or phenomena, not physical elements. As I see it, the realm of Vibration and Magnetism is itself a borderline between the potentiality of Sacred Space and the world of physical manifestation. It comes right between the first stirrings of One-becoming-Two (in the Brow Chakra) and the first physical element, Air (in the Heart Chakra).

As I was contemplating this whole subject, in preparation for the first writing of this book (in 2002), a friend sent me an article about the Mayan Calendar as explained by Carlos Barrios, a historian, anthropologist, and Mayan ceremonial priest in Guatemala. In the article, he talks about changes that will come to Earth beginning at the Winter Solstice of 2012. The Mayan Calendar shows that date as the start of a new era called the World of the Fifth Sun.

This is from the article:[2]

> Mr. Barrios said the emerging era of the Fifth Sun will call attention to a much-overlooked element. Whereas the four traditional elements of earth, air, fire and water have dominated various epochs in the past, there will be a fifth element to reckon with in the time of the Fifth Sun: ether.
>
> The dictionary defines ether as the rarefied element thought to fill the upper regions of space, the Heavens. Ether is a medium that permeates all space and transmits waves of energy in a wide range of

frequencies, from cell phones to human auras. What is "ethereal" is related to the regions beyond earth: the heavens.

Ether—the element of the Fifth Sun—is celestial, and lacking in material substance, but is no less real than wood, wind, flame, stone or flesh.

"Within the context of ether there can be a fusion of the polarities," Mr. Barrios said. "No more darkness or light in the people, but an uplifted fusion."

Hmmm … the end of duality! Isn't that really the goal of Usui's "method to achieve personal perfection"—by achieving true Self-realization? This coming end-of-duality seems also to have been anticipated by Nakazono-sensei. In his writings on kototama, he presented three principles governing the manifestation of life (from *a priori* to *a posteriori*). Our current civilization, he said, is guided by two of these principles together—Amatsu Kanagi ("the order of human expression based on the perception of the physical senses") and Amatsu Sugaso ("the order of human expression based on the perception of the spiritual senses")—and he said this about the third principle, Amatsu Futonolito ("the complete order of expression of human life"),[3] which was hidden from humanity about ten thousand years ago:

> Once it [Futonolito] was hidden, humanity could no longer realize the complete content of its inner capacities. We only had the Amatsu Kanagi and Amatsu Sugaso viewpoints to guide us.
>
> If we know and practice Amatsu Futonolito, we can clearly see the contents of the other two principles. The reverse is not true. If Futonolito is hidden, we have nowhere to turn for the truth.[4]

Mr. Barrios is talking about a new awareness of an etheric element, which will allow us to reconcile all dualities in a transformational way. Notice that the article says the new era "will call attention to a much-overlooked element." The element is already here, already within us (and, like the aspects of Reiki, has always been within us, I suppose). What will make the new era different is our conscious awakening to the etheric element and its properties. Perhaps we don't even have to wait until 2012—we can begin awakening now!

So, now we have:

Earth—at the Root Chakra

Water—at the Sacral Chakra

Tree—at the navel

Fire—at the Solar Plexus

Air—at the Heart Chakra

Ether—at the Throat Chakra.

Next let's look at an empowerment procedure based on my aware-ness of these energies and the realization of the human body as a miniature of the greater Universe. I call it the "You Are The Universe!" Empowerment.

"You Are The Universe!"—An Empowerment

Until I spent some time with a Reiki teacher in Singapore, I had never seen or heard of, or even thought of, giving a Reiki empowerment to a reclining recipient. But that was the way Catherine gave empower-ments and it made sense to me, just because a reclining recipient could be more fully relaxed than a sitting recipient. So, thanks to Catherine, the following Reiki empowerment is done with the recipient lying down.

This empowerment uses a concept known in Chi-gung as the Micro-cosmic Orbit: the idea that in the personal microcosm, there is a natu-ral orbit of energy down the front of the body (from Crown to Root) and up the back (from Root to Crown). On the front, I also like to incorporate the Usui Stone Method (described in Chapter 8).

I start with the recipient lying face up. First I smooth down the aura. Then I place the jade at the Heart Chakra. I rest two fingers on it and intone (either mentally or aloud) the Harmony kotodama, to invoke the aspects of Light, Heaven, Harmony. Then I place the quartz at the Brow Chakra, resting the fingers and intoning the Connection kotodama, to invoke Love, Oneness. Then I place the citrine at the Throat Chakra, resting the fingers and intoning the Focus kotodama, to invoke Power, Focus. Usually I tone each kotodama a few times, until I feel a strong connection with the spirit of it. And I add a fourth stone, amethyst, at the Crown—using the Empowerment kotodama with it.

Then I position myself at the head and proceed through what might appear to be a basic Reiki treatment. However, as I place my hands in each position, I am concentrating a particular awareness there. Here is the order of placement, and the corresponding awareness for each position:

Forehead/Brow: Greeting the person by name, connecting, acknowledging our Oneness (intoning Connection kotodama). Also greeting the Reiki in the body, and giving thanks for the empowerment that is about to occur.

Crown: Opening, as fully as possible, this gateway to Source (intoning Empowerment kotodama). Thanking the energy, inviting it to fill and overflow everything. (And, here's a good question: Is it filling from *outside,* through the Crown ... or is it filling from *inside,* through a Source-dimension within every wave-particle of our physical being?)

SOURCE
DESCENDS—

CREATING:
((SACRED))
((SPACE))

Temples:
Ears:
Back of Head:

Intoning Harmony
kotodama—

which
DESCENDS—

CREATING:
duality, polarity,
yin & yang,
Vibration,
Magnetism

Throat:
(little fingers
resting on clavicle)

Intoning Focus
kotodama—

Incorporating Ether into
Vibration and Magnetism

which
DESCEND—
giving birth to All That Is,
through the elements of:

((AIR))
(BREATH / SOUL)
(SKY)

Heart:
(fingertips of one hand
meeting heel of other,
extending from clavicle
downward)

Intoning Empowerment
kotodama—

(the vibration is more
materialized here than
at the Crown)

Now the person brings up the hands in gassho. I put one of my hands on either side of theirs, in the aura, and let the energy flow, with the intent of centering the Universe there and opening the conduit from the Heart through the arms and hands.

Now their hands go back alongside the body, and I move from the head to the side and continue moving downward:

((AIR))
(BREATH / SOUL)
(SKY)

DESCENDS,
BECOMING—

Solar Plexus:
(extending from bottom
of sternum to navel)

((FIRE))
(SUN)
(day, bright,
active, yang)

Intoning Harmony
kotodama—

(the vibration is more
materialized here than in the
head: Fire instead of Light)

DESCENDS,
BECOMING—

Navel:
(both palms
directly over it)

((TREE))
(receives light,
transforms it
to water)

No kotodama here—

(bridge between Fire
and Water)

DESCENDS,
BECOMING—

Sacral Chakra:
(both palms directly
over it; then one on
each hip bone)

((WATER))
(MOON)
(night, dark, passive,
reflective, yin)

Intoning Connection
kotodama—
Oneness, Love

(the vibration is more
materialized here than
at the Forehead/Brow)

DESCENDS,
BECOMING—

Knees:
Ankles:
Soles of Feet:

((EARTH))
(EARTH)
(grounding)

Intoning Focus kotodama—

(the vibration is more
materialized here than
at the Throat)

Now, when the person feels ready, we do the back side, working up from the Root Chakra (*read this sequence from bottom up*):

SOURCE	**Crown:**	Intoning Empowerment kotodama— (vibration more subtle than at the Heart)
	ASCENDS, BECOMING—	
((SACRED)) (SPACE)	**Back and Sides of Head:**	Intoning Harmony kotodama— (vibration more subtle than at Solar Plexus)
	ASCENDS, BECOMING—	
Magnetism, Vibration, polarity, duality	**Back of Throat:** (5th Cervical vertebra)	Intoning Focus kotodama— (vibration more subtle than at Root Chakra)
	ASCENDS, BECOMING—	
((AIR)) (BREATH) (SOUL) (SKY)	**Heart:**	Intoning Empowerment kotodama—
	ASCENDS, BECOMING—	
((FIRE)) (consumes and transforms Tree)	**Solar Plexus:**	Intoning Harmony kotodama—
	ASCENDS, BECOMING—	
((TREE)) (takes Water from Earth)	**Back of Navel:**	No kotodama here— (bridge between Water and Fire)

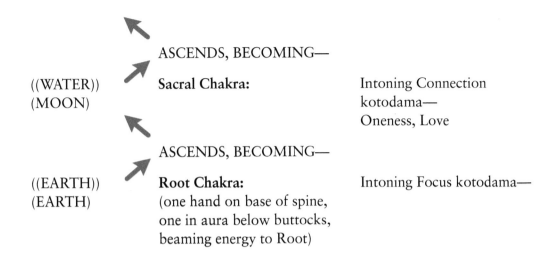

ASCENDS, BECOMING—

((WATER))   **Sacral Chakra:**   Intoning Connection
(MOON)   kotodama—
                                              Oneness, Love

ASCENDS, BECOMING—

((EARTH))   **Root Chakra:**   Intoning Focus kotodama—
(EARTH)   (one hand on base of spine,
             one in aura below buttocks,
             beaming energy to Root)

You might like to use this procedure the first time someone comes to you for Reiki. It's a thorough treatment/empowerment, and it allows maximum relaxation of the recipient.

Possibly what gives greatest effectiveness and empowers us the most is accurate understanding: having a concept that aligns with reality. My perception of Reiki has transformed enormously since my first contact with it. At this writing, my "You Are The Universe!" concept seems very workable and fitting to me. I've come to see increasingly that all the elements of Reiki—in fact, all the energies of the greater Universe—have been within us from the time of our conception in Spirit. There is nothing external to us, not even the Source; it only seems that way until our awareness reaches a certain point. I believe empowerment is a matter of conscious awareness.

After the "You Are The Universe!" empowerment, I give the person a demonstration and a written description of the self-treatment. Then they can start giving themselves Reiki. Many people begin receiving weekly Reiju then; and some decide to go through the official levels of training.

Reiki and Theta Waves

We've been taught to connect with different aspects of Reiki by using certain symbols and/or kotodama, but what about our energetic condition at the time of doing this? How can we knowingly put ourselves in an optimal vibratory state for maximizing the effectiveness of Reiki?

Obviously, it's best to be still and calm and somehow meditative—but can we be more specific than that? Can we adjust our vibratory frequency to an optimal range?

The study of brain waves (as measured by electroencephalograph) has led scientists to define five particular ranges of brain activity, each one associated with characteristic behaviors or effects, as follows:[5]

- Delta (approx. 0.5–4 cycles per second): the predominant realm of human brain activity from birth to age two; after that time, Delta is the state of deep, dreamless sleep, in which the concept of individual/ego dissolves completely—and so do awareness and memory; Delta can also be used for deep, hypnotic programming.

- Theta (approx. 4–8 cycles per second): This is where we spend most of our time from age two to six—the realm where we access intuition, instant healing, accelerated learning, and the feeling of Oneness-with-All; also the brain wave of the shamanic state (it's no accident that shamanic drumming is done at frequencies of 4–7 beats per second). Theta is also used in hypnotherapy.

- Alpha (approx. 8–12 cycles per second): We move primarily into this realm from age six to twelve; it's a relaxed, meditative state, the awareness of "self" and consciousness.

- Beta (approx. 12–35 cycles per second): We begin to show sustained periods at this frequency around age twelve; it's the realm of the highly focused, individual ego, where most adults spend most of their time.

- Gamma (above 35 cycles per second): This is the realm of "peak performance"; the state of consciousness that some people have referred to as "the zone."

From this information, it seems that a brain-wave frequency in the Theta range is the best for any kind of healing, including Reiki. When people's brain waves have been monitored while doing Reiki, though, they usually measure in the Alpha range. Clearly, the lower-frequency Theta waves are more helpful in realizing our Oneness, helping us to "get out of our own way" and let the high-frequency vibrations of Reiki do their job. So—how can we intentionally put our brain waves in the Theta range?

How to Achieve Theta

I discovered this quite by "accident" one night, years ago—when I was not even aware of the different brain-wave states. I had agreed to do distant Reiki with someone (my Reiki teacher!) late at night ... and had fallen asleep before the appointed time. I awoke in the middle of the night—not even knowing what time it was—remembering that I had to do the Reiki.

I sat up in bed, barely awake, and attempted to do it. I could not even get my eyes fully open; the lids were nearly closed, in fact. I could hardly hold a mental focus for more than a few moments. I tried a few times, and then simply mustered as much intent as I could that Reiki be received by my teacher at the time we had agreed on. Then I lay back down in the bed and was immediately asleep.

My Reiki teacher called on the phone the next day to tell me in detail of the most wonderful Reiki she had received through me; it had been a spectacularly transforming experience for her! I was quite surprised, to say the least—and too cowardly to tell her how things had gone at my end. (Deb, if you're reading this now, at last you know!) But it was a great lesson for me about doing Reiki. It taught me, first of all, that intent is more effective than procedure; *and that I did my best Reiki when I was half-asleep!*

What had struck me most about my experience that night was my deep state of drowsiness, and the nearly-closed position of my eyes. I kept feeling there was something important in that. So I began, when doing Reiki after that time, holding my eyes intentionally in that position. I would let them close, almost but not quite all the way, and I would un-focus the vision—and I noticed an immediately enhanced flow of Reiki!

Simply letting the eyes drop almost but not quite closed put me immediately in a deeply meditative state. There was a slight feeling of drowsiness, but it was easy to stay right on the edge of it, on the border between consciousness and unconsciousness. I've been doing Reiki this way ever since—and it was years before I encountered the scientific data that confirm why it works so well.

There's great information on the Web regarding Theta brain waves and their effectiveness in instantaneous healing, accelerated learning, deliberate creation, and the relationship of DNA to all this.

Some links you may find interesting:

www.bethcoleman.net/theta.html
www.risingsunhealing.com/artDNAActivation.html
www.thetahealing.com

Vianna Stibal, of thetahealing.com, has developed her own healing system and published *ThetaHealing: Go Up and Seek God, Go Up and Work With God.*[6] Vianna has her own way of getting into Theta vibration. In classes given by her, she says, people's brain waves were measured going into Theta immediately upon holding the intention of going up and seeking God. She also says some interesting things about Theta waves and Gamma waves working together: that, in emergency situations, the brain has been measured going back and forth between Theta and Gamma vibrations, skipping everything in between. And she feels that this Theta-Gamma-alternating state is the very best for bringing about instantaneous healing.

Heal Yourself, Heal the World!

Possibly the greatest thing Reiki reveals to us is the Oneness of all life. We come to see that healing ourselves is one of the greatest contributions we can make to the good of all. We live in an infinite hologram, in which the whole infinity of creation is complete in every wave-particle! It's not just "One for all, and all for one," it's "One *is* all, and all *is* one." That means we cannot possibly heal ourselves *without* healing (at least a little bit) everything else, too. If that ain't magic, it's the next best thing!

Of course, being human, we like to think we can improve even on magic. Instead of spending *all* our time on self-healing, we like also to give healing to each other. We enjoy the feeling of giving and receiving gifts. And there is something very powerful in the giving and receiving. A gift, given and received with love, is often so much better than anything we can do for ourselves.

It's very easy, and very rewarding, to "give healing/awakening" to any list of particular individuals, every day as we empower and heal ourselves. The individuals can be people, relationships, animals, plants, machines, events, fundamental elements, geographic regions, planets and galaxies whirling through the cosmos—anything imaginable. We cannot force the healing, but we can offer it.

A version of this practice is described in the "You Are The Universe!" self-treatment, in Chapter 3. With a little experimentation and reflection, I'm sure your intuition will provide the most fitting method for you (which is likely to change over time).

For several years, my usual method was to use the basic Reiju procedure, preceded by the breathing exercise described in Chapter 4 (see "An Energy Exercise of My Own"), incorporating my version of the Reiki Concepts. I lived near some protected ocean pools, and my favorite way of doing Reiju was while standing in them (with the water at about knee-level). I would bring my hands together in gassho; I would let my eyelids drop almost but not quite closed (see "Reiki and Theta Waves," just above) . . . and the following prayer would echo through my mind:

> Dear Infinite Source, Thank You, thank you, thank you, filling and overflowing, NOW, from within, every wave-particle of every be-ing,[7] everywhere, for the greatest awareness, greatest em-pow-er-ment! And par-tic-u-lar-ly, this dear planet Earth, for the greatest peace, and wholeness, and well-be-ing. And par-tic-u-lar-ly, all Ether [feeling it in the Throat Chakra] . . . all Air [feeling it in the Heart Chakra] . . . all Fire [feeling it in the Solar Plexus Chakra] . . . all Tree [feeling it in the navel] . . . all Water [feeling it in the Sacral Chakra] . . . all Earth [feeling it in the Root Chakra]. And par-tic-u-lar-ly, each individual named on our Reiju List and our

Healing Circle List[8] for this day: [e.g.] Year 2008, December, Friday, twenty-sixth day; to be perceived by each at the most beneficial time, for the greatest awareness, greatest em-pow-er-ment, greatest Self-realization.

Then I would do the breathing exercise. Then the Reiju, and final thanks. The whole process would take twenty minutes or less and would leave me feeling wonderfully energized (while helping to heal and empower all other beings!).

Once you've worked for a time with any of these techniques for directing energy, I think you'll find, as I have, that less and less technique is required. My methods almost always get simpler—until they eventually converge on the single point of Intent. Once we really know how to do something, we learn to do it without doing it! We learn simply to witness what is already done—and that *everything* is already done.

All Hands Report for Duty!

When giving Reiki, it's not necessary to limit ourselves to using only two hands! People become so relaxed and peaceful, I don't like to disturb them at all—to get my hands under their head, for instance—and instead I merely "feel" a pair of "spirit" hands going there. In addition to not disturbing the person, this effectively puts four hands on them instead of two—doubling the Reiki! The physical hands don't require my attention, so I can easily focus on the "spirit" hands.

Likewise, instead of disturbing the person to turn over, I often use "spirit" hands on their back to mirror the positions of my physical hands on the front. Directing Reiki from both sides at the same time, in this way, seems especially beneficial. Even beyond the enhanced

Reiki, an extra benefit is that people don't have to lie face-down, which is uncomfortable for many (whether using a face-holder or turning the neck to lay the head flat).

Another excellent use of this is to give Reiki simultaneously to widely separated areas of the body: the crown and the soles of feet, for instance; or shoulders and ankles; etc.

Using more than one set of hands in this way not only enhances the effectiveness of Reiki, it makes treatment time shorter than otherwise!

Part Four

Beyond Reiki

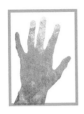

Chapter 11

Johrei

Purifying Spirit

In the fall of 1999, a few months after receiving my third-level Reiki Attunements, I became interested in Johrei, the "purifying spirit" energy developed by Mokichi Okada. I happened to see an ad for an introductory presentation of Johrei at a nearby food co-op. I wanted to see how Johrei compared with Reiki; but, due to a previous commitment, I was unable to attend the presentation. I figured there would be another one eventually, and maybe I could go to it.

A week or so later, I was exchanging Reiki with another Reiki teacher—just barely starting to give her Reiki—when she said, "You're doing something more than just Reiki, aren't you?"

If so, I wasn't conscious of it. "Like what?" I said.

"Like Johrei," she said.

This really got my attention; it seemed quite a coincidence to be hearing this so shortly after my wanting to attend the Johrei presentation. I asked what she knew about Johrei, and why she felt she was receiving it through me. She said she knew nothing about it, that the word had simply come into her mind!

This was much too coincidental for me to ignore. The next day I called the food co-op and got a phone number for the person who had made the Johrei presentation. When I spoke with her, she told me there was a local Johrei group that met once a week, and I was welcome to attend and receive Johrei.

I began doing so, and immediately knew I wanted to learn to give Johrei. I was asked to receive Johrei twenty times before taking the eighteen-hour training course. I did so, then took the course (which was mostly on the history and spiritual teachings of Johrei's founder, Mokichi Okada), becoming a member of Johrei Fellowship in the spring of 2000.[1]

Since I first began learning about Johrei, I couldn't help noticing many parallels with Reiki. First of all, the word *rei* in the name: It's the same as in *Rei-ki,* meaning "spirit"; and *joh* means "purifying." *Joh-rei* = "purifying spirit." Its founder, Mokichi Okada, was born in 1882, barely a generation after Usui—and both were living in Tokyo in the 1920s.

What struck me most of all was Okada's use of Dai Ko Myo, the Usui Master symbol. The Johrei calligraphy sometimes called "White Light"—which has been used for decades on altars in Johrei Centers and in the homes of members—is composed of five Japanese kanji, the first three being Dai Ko Myo.[2] In the calligraphy as usually seen, they don't appear the same as in the Reiki symbol, only because the calligraphy is done in a cursive style of writing, which looks very different. At left, I've put the Johrei calligraphy in a more basic style, to make the Dai Ko Myo recognizable.

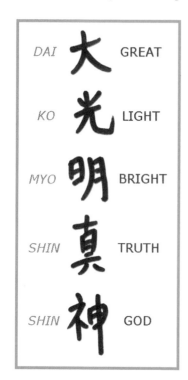

DAI	大	GREAT
KO	光	LIGHT
MYO	明	BRIGHT
SHIN	真	TRUTH
SHIN	神	GOD

Johrei "White Light"
(calligraphy by Mio)

Mokichi Okada was a businessman and artist, and a member of the spiritual group Omoto Kyo, before founding Johrei. The story of his transformation is quite remarkable. He was a member of Omoto Kyo when, in December 1926 (just nine months after the passing of Mikao Usui), he began receiving spontaneous transmissions of spiritual information. He spoke them to his wife, who wrote them down as he dictated. This continued for three months. The information was about all aspects of life, on Earth and in the spirit worlds, and included much about the very ancient history of Japan.

At some point Okada came to understand that the information, and the new direction his life was taking, came from the Bodhisattva Kannon (the one associated with the Reiki Connection symbol). At least one person saw the spirit

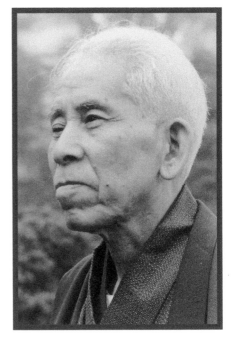

Mokichi Okada
Image courtesy Nakahashi Sensei/ Temple Light from the East (www.lux-oriens.com.br).

of Kannon following Okada around; and later a photo was taken in which a ghostly image of Kannon appears hovering above Okada!

Eventually Okada, with instruction from Kannon, developed a way of working with the purifying energy he would later call Johrei. In 1935 he officially inaugurated the Japan Kannon Society, which in later years became Sekai Kyusei Kyo and Johrei Fellowship.

Okada was the Spiritual Leader *(Meishu)* of the Kannon Society, and members began calling him simply Meishu-sama.[3] His teachings included the spiritual nature of food and the importance of growing it naturally, with no artificial additives; also, the raising of one's vibration through appreciating the beauty of Nature and through making and experiencing works of art, as well as through the transmission of Johrei energy.

I've read, on the Web sites of two Reiki teachers (neither one affiliated with Johrei), that Johrei uses Reiju as an empowerment procedure. This has not been my experience, and I don't know where they got this idea. (I wrote to ask and received no response from either of them.) Johrei empowerment involves the wearing of a physical object called a "sacred focal point" *(ohikari)*. It is worn on a cord around the neck, under the clothing, at the level of the heart.

Over the years, the focal points have taken different forms. The earliest ones were simply a calligraphy done by Okada on a sheet of paper, then the paper was folded several times and placed in a small cloth bag. In my experience with Johrei Fellowship, the focal point is still a calligraphy but the container is a small titanium disk. An individual guardian spirit is assigned to each focal point, which is then presented to the new member in a short ceremony. The actual empowerment, however—at least in my experience—is done with no procedure except a simple prayer.

Okada's own description of how this worked was as follows: He was connected to Kannon by a spiritual cord; the divine light of Kannon came to him through this cord, manifesting as a ball of light in his abdomen; and, by merely writing the ideogram for "light" on a paper and giving the paper to someone (to be folded up and worn in a pouch hung from the neck), that person was connected, by a spiritual cord, to the infinite divine light of Kannon, via Okada. This is the light that is transmitted as Johrei. Okada said that, in his making of the focal points, not even a prayer was involved. He simply wrote the ideograms, as fast as he could—and he could write five hundred of them in an hour!

In the early days, the calligraphy done by Okada for the focal point was Dai Ko Myo. Later, for a time, some focal points were Dai Ko Myo, some were Ko Myo, and some were just Ko (which is what the Johrei Fellowship now uses in all its focal points).

I realize it could be simply coincidence that both Usui and Okada used Dai Ko Myo as a symbol of empowerment in their methods of working with subtle energy; Dai Ko Myo is rather ubiquitous in Japan, after all. Still, so many coincidences made me wonder if there had been any personal contact between the two men.

Unlike the situation with Usui and Reiki, a detailed written history of Johrei has been kept by Okada's followers. Okada himself left many volumes of writings (though few of them have been translated to English, and his family has kept much of the material secret from everyone else). In the Johrei material I've read, I've not seen any mention of a link between Usui and Okada; likewise, the archives of Omoto Kyo record no such connection. But I was told of one personal testimony of exactly that. A daughter of Mrs. Kimiko Koyama (a past President of the Usui Gakkai) reportedly said that her mother knew both Okada and Onisaburo Deguchi (the leader of Omoto Kyo), and that both were students of Mikao Usui. I have no way to verify or deny it myself—but it does seem reasonable.

In any case, there's no denying the importance of Dai Ko Myo in Johrei, as in Reiki: Dai Ko Myo, Great Light Sun-and-Moon. In Reiki, we've seen that the energy of Fire (Sun) is associated with Symbol #2, Sei He Ki; and that the energy of Water (Moon) is associated with Symbol #3, Hon Sha Ze Sho Nen. And we see, in the Reiki "empowerment" symbol—#4, Dai Ko Myo—that both Fire (Sun) and Water (Moon) are present, together, in Myo. Mokichi Okada made it very clear that, in Johrei, the joining-together of these seemingly opposite energies—Fire and Water—was itself a crucial element. He felt that Fire-and-Water (Sun-and-Moon) together were what created the divine light of Kannon, which Okada passed on to others via his Johrei focal points.

In his understanding, the importance of this Fire-and-Water combination from Kannon was linked to the very nature of health in the human body. Okada said the two most important organs in the body were the heart and lungs, in that order. The heart absorbed the spirit of Fire, he said, and the lungs absorbed the spirit of Water. A third energy was also important, and that was Earth. Okada said the Earth element was provided by the stomach, which he viewed as the third most important human organ. In fact, he called these three elements—Fire, Water, and Earth—the very essence of the human body. And, he said, the only rational way to heal the body was by using these three elements.

He described the disease process as beginning with the accumulation of "clouds" on the spiritual body. If these clouds were not removed, they would become toxins in the physical body; and these solidified toxins were the cause of all disease. He felt that Johrei was especially effective at removing both spiritual clouds and physical toxins—because of its divine light, created by the conjunction of Fire-and-Water. Johrei provided an abundance of that; and the third essential energy, Earth, was provided by the human body itself, specifically the stomach.

We see, then, that Reiki and Johrei involve the same subtle energies, but their presence comes about in different ways. With Reiki, we learn to "become" Earth energy, and then Heaven energy (Fire/Sun), and then Oneness (itself associated with Water/Moon—and Kannon). With Johrei, the combination of Fire-and-Water (Sun-and-Moon) comes to us from Kannon, and combines with the spirit of Earth, present already in the physical body. (It should be noted that the body also contains its own measure of Fire-and-Water, but that is minuscule compared to the amount we receive through Johrei/Kannon.) Okada believed that the *order* in which these energies combined was crucial to the effectiveness of Johrei; that it was essential for the Fire-and-Water combination to arrive first, and then to combine with the Earth element of the physical body.

Here's something quite intriguing to me: Okada also said that:

- the spirit of Fire = oxygen
- the spirit of Water = hydrogen
- the spirit of Earth = nitrogen

Fire, Water, and Earth made up his list of elements essential for life; no mention of Air. But, how do we take in oxygen, hydrogen, and nitrogen? By breathing the Air! In fact, most of what we're breathing is nitrogen, the spirit of Earth!

This also explains how "breatharians" and others can indeed live without eating what the rest of us call food. They are taking in the crucial three elements just by breathing! Mostly, they're breathing the spirit of Earth—and usually they get a lot more Fire element by sungazing. And, of course, the Water element is obtained by drinking water (because the amount of hydrogen, that is Water-spirit, in the air is barely measurable).[4]

Johrei Energy

My first impression, on receiving Johrei, was that it was more powerful than Reiki. I've come to believe that's not necessarily the case, and it seems that both energies can bring about the same results. They do seem different in character, though. Reiki seems more gentle and balanced and rounded to me; Johrei feels sharper and more concentrated. I believe it's this sharpness that I first equated with increased power (plus the fact of it being a "new" energy to me then).

Johrei was originally given hands-on, similar to Reiki. Then, at some point, the procedure was changed to "beaming" with one hand, due to governmental concerns about physical contact. Now the standard procedure—and everything in Johrei is much more standardized than in Reiki—is to sit facing the recipient (also seated) and beam Johrei to the front of the body; then the recipient turns around and Johrei is beamed to the back. The entire session normally lasts only twenty to thirty minutes.

Okada believed that our world was heading for an imminent purification by Fire, and that only by giving and receiving sufficient amounts of Johrei could we purify ourselves enough to survive and mitigate the coming fiery events on Earth.

It's interesting to me that, historically, Johrei appeared shortly after Usui developed his Reiki method. In recent years the awareness and popularity of Reiki has mushroomed globally, and I can't help wondering, "Is Johrei next?" Is there truly something in its nature that makes it the most appropriate energy for the times we are now entering?

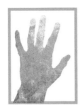

Chapter 12

Other Voices,
Other Rooms

Meishu-sama talked a lot about humanity's emergence from the Age of Night into the Daylight Age. He even decreed that the Daylight Age began on a particular date in 1934. Of course, there have been (and continue to be) countless other voices heralding this New Age—and it seems we are undeniably into it. Our awareness is growing by such quantum leaps, in fact, that Meishu-sama's messianic vision of Johrei— dare I say it!—looks a bit isolated and outdated. This is meant not to reduce Johrei in the slightest, only to point out that we're in the midst of a global Self-awakening, the enormity of which could not have been imagined by Meishu-sama. There are so many voices arising now, from so many rooms, and they're all saying the same thing: Awaken to Reality, awaken to the Truth of Self—whether by way of Johrei, or Reiki, or any of ten thousand other methods!

We must all awaken and "save" ourselves. Part of the awakening is to realize that there is no external messiah of any sort. There is no external *anything!* What we see as external are merely projections— flickering images of light on a movie screen—of aspects of Self. And there is only one Self! All is One: One is All: The Great Hologram.

All healing/awakening, regardless of any method or technique involved, is simply the unification of the Universal and the personal. This unification has been the true state of existence always, but we've gone through a period of fooling ourselves by projecting *false* images—of separation, duality, conflict—and now it's time for the return of Truth. And nothing will stop it.

For me, the first seeds of conscious awakening were planted over thirty years ago—when I read a book by Jane Roberts, and a book on Raja Yoga, and the books of Paul Brunton. Then, for many years, I worked on discovering myself through writing—while reading countless other books on spiritual awakening and practicing many systems of formal meditation. When it seemed I had reached the end of writing—sick of words!—Reiki came along. Eventually I recognized that Reiki was indeed my preferred form of meditation, and I said goodbye to the others.

Along the way, Macrobiotics and Johrei found me and have incorporated themselves into me. More recently, my understanding of the reality of Oneness continues to grow deeper roots, thanks greatly to the teachings of Dr. Hew Len and Joe Vitale (and Dr. Len's modern version of the ancient Hawai'ian practice of Ho'oponopono), Joel S. Goldsmith, Mikoto Nakazono, and Frederick Bailes. Most recently, it was the words of Bailes[1] that really brought home to me, at a deeper level than before, how—*yes!*—*all healing/awakening, whatever method or technique may be involved, is simply the unification of the Universal and the personal.* That is to say, in a single word, *Rei-ki.* And I find, whatever other concepts and practices I have come to incorporate, the conscious daily connection of Reiki is still the most nurturing and satisfying to me.

Thank you so very much, dear Usui-sensei, Usui-sama!

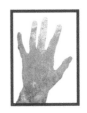

Glossary

dojo: "Place of the Way." A training center. A place where one goes to learn and practice a Way *(do)* of life.

gakkai: An association for educational purposes, a Society or Club; and sometimes used as a front for religious activities.

gassho: Bringing the palms of the hands together in a "prayer position." It means, literally, "two hands coming together," and it has a centering and connecting effect in the body.

hara: Belly.

kanji: Pictograms of Chinese origin, used in writing the Japanese language.

kenkyukai: An association for research purposes, though sometimes used as a front for religious activities.

kotodama (or kototama): "Spirit words" or "spirit language." The "word of God," which brings the manifest world into being.

Okuden: The second level of Reiki training (meaning "Inner Teachings" or "The Deep Inside").

Reiju: Literally, "giving Spirit"—an energetic "empowerment" procedure, taught by Mikao Usui, for awakening one's awareness of Reiki. According to some of Usui's students, it was taken from Tendai Buddhism.

seiza: "Proper sitting posture" (see photo in "Usui Shoden," in Chapter 4).

sensei: A term of respect commonly used by students in reference to their teacher. Literally it denotes a pioneer or pathfinder, meaning "one who goes before."

Shinpiden: The third level of Reiki training (meaning "Mystery Teachings" or "The Mystery").

Shoden: The first level of Reiki training (meaning "First Teachings" or "The Entrance").

tanden: Literally, "red field"; commonly translated as "elixir field" (referring to a field in which the "elixir of life" is planted). The body has three of these fields: one centered in the head, one in the chest or solar plexus, and one in the abdomen. In Reiki, the word "tanden" has generally been used in reference not to these fields but to a single *point*, below the navel. (See "The Tanden and the One Point," in Chapter 3.)

waka: Native poems.

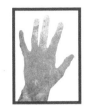

Notes

Introduction

1. Author of *O-Sensei: A View of Mikao Usui* (China: David King, 2006).
2. Author of *Reiki: The Legacy of Dr. Usui* (Twin Lakes: Lotus Press, 1998) and other books.
3. This came from Mr. Hiroshi Doi, a member of the URR Gakkai, who was featured at the first Usui Reiki Ryoho International conference, in Vancouver, B.C., Canada (1999). Mr. Doi subsequently published *Iyashino Gendai Reiki-ho* or *Modern Reiki Method for Healing* (Canada: Fraser Journal Publishing, 2000).
4. The names I've used for the Reiki degrees—The Entrance, The Deep Inside, and The Mystery—were the translations presented by Hiroshi Doi at the first Usui Reiki Ryoho International (URRI) conference, in 1999. I've since been told, by Dave King, that the more common translations are, respectively: First Teachings, Inner Teachings, and Mystery Teachings.

Chapter 1

1. Historically, this has been the conventional view, that heavenly or universal or spiritual energy comes to us from above. I've come to believe, however, that our most direct connection with such energy is from within; that our Source is truly and literally within every physical wave-particle of us, and that Reiki awakens us to that connection.
2. See www.asunam.com/life_of_mikao_usui.htm.
3. See "Three Reiki Students in the Year 2001," later in Chapter 1. My communication with Taggart King has been by email.

4. This was confirmed by Dave King's information from a Buddhist nun called Tenon-in, who was a student and associate of Usui for years.

5. The manual given to students in the Usui Gakkai also contains *waka*, specifically, ones written by the Meiji Emperor (which are called *gyosei*). These are not the waka Usui used; his were chosen because they contained certain *kotodama* (sacred sounds). In contrast, the information from Dave King (no relation to Taggart) is that Usui had no written manual until 1925, when Dr. Hayashi—one of Usui's final students (and a naval surgeon)—was asked to create one.

6. In one of his Reiki manuals, which he sent me.

7. See www.asunam.com/life_of_mikao_usui.htm.

8. Andrew Bowling is an English teacher of Reiki, and an associate of Chris Marsh. See www.threshold.ca/AndrewBowling/Usui.html.

9. Both Dave King and Chris Marsh, who have learned from different students of Mikao Usui, have referred to the use of "Usui-do" by the students. However, Dave has also said: "We later found out that the preferred reading of 'Usui-Do' was 'Usui-no-michi' (with an identical meaning)."

10. According to Dave King, the kanji in question here are *gakkai mouke*, which he says can be interpreted "to mean whatever you like since it lacks any context as written. One interpretation is simply that 'he opened a dojo.' Doi-san interprets it as 'he founded the URR Gakkai.'"

11. Toshihiro (a.k.a. Toshitoro) Eguchi was the teacher of Yuji Onuki, the man who taught Dave King and Melissa Riggall a form of Usui-do in 1971, in Morocco.

12. A Buddhist nun who passed away in 2005 at the age of 107, Tenon-in (a.k.a. Mariko) was with Mikao Usui, as a student and associate, almost every day from 1920 to 1926.

13. *Jikiden* can be translated as "direct transmission of mysteries or skill."

14. This connection with Usui-sensei was mentioned by a daughter of Mrs. Kimiko Koyama, a past President of the Usui Gakkai. Kimiko herself knew Deguchi and Okada.

15. Some people interpret this to mean just a large number, not exactly defined;

others believe it can be taken literally, but that it includes those taught by students of Usui.

16. Excerpts copyright © 1971–2005 Dave King and Melissa Riggall; reprinted by permission. See www.threshold.ca/usui-do/stories.shtml#lbl4.

[17.] Mount Hiei-zan, northeast of Kyoto. On top of the mountain is Enryakuji, a Tendai Buddhist temple, one of the main spiritual centers of Japan. The temple on Mount Kurama was a "branch" of this temple, and Usui normally attended the main temple, Enryakuji, on Hiei-zan.

[18.] This was his first "seat of learning" in Tokyo. Notice that the date is the same as recorded on Usui's gravestone (in some translations, at least) as the founding of the URR Gakkai!

[19.] According to Dave King, Eguchi wanted to chant a prayer (called "Koumiyou Kagan"), which he had received from Nishida, at the start of each meeting; and the "blessing" was a ceremony called Denju.

20. The term "Shinto kotodama" seems nebulous, at best. The oldest koto-tama (a variable English spelling for the same word) system I know of was the one taught by Mikoto Nakazono; then there are the much more recent systems, developed by Omoto Kyo (Deguchi) and Aikido (Ueshiba and others). Chronologically, Shinto arose between the two—but there is really no definable *system* of Shinto kotodama, only the existence of certain Shinto prayers and poems that are perceived to contain koto-dama. So, the real origin of the Usui kotodama seems to be another Reiki mystery.

21. It has long been said that Dr. Hayashi was a Christian Methodist, and this was confirmed by one of his students, Mrs. Yamaguchi (who passed away in 2003). Other sources have said that Hayashi practiced the Soto Zen religion. It's quite possible that he was involved in both; such a thing is not uncommon in Japan.

22. Dave King, on the other hand, says Hayashi *did* learn the complete Usui-do system from Usui—a system involving no energetic empowerments!

23. Another Reiki mystery: Ms. Takata was recorded, in 1979, saying that Dr. Hayashi had taught her exactly what he learned from Usui, and that

she taught exactly what she had learned from Hayashi, with no changes. This mirrors precisely what Dave King and Melissa Riggall were told by another student of Hayashi's, a Mr. Tatsumi: that he had been taught exactly what Usui taught Hayashi—and yet the teachings of Tatsumi and Takata were remarkably different, even down to the naming of the system ("Usui-do" and "Usui Shiki Ryoho," respectively).

24. This is disputed by Dr. Barbara Ray, another student of Takata, who claims that she, Barbara, is the true successor, and that Takata taught her Reiki secrets that were given to no one else. She calls these "The Intact Master Keys of Reiki," claims that authentic Usui Reiki consists of seven degrees, and that these "Intact Master Keys" have been held only by Usui, Hayashi, Takata, and herself. In 1980 she founded her own organization, The American Reiki Association, Inc. (now called The Radiance Technique International Association, Inc.).

Chapter 2

1. Copyright © 2002 Dave King. The Japanese kanji and their pronunciations, plus Dave's explanations, can be seen at www.threshold.ca/reiki/Usui-Gainen.html.

2. *Gassho* is bringing the palms of the hands together in a "prayer position." It means, literally, "two hands coming together," and it has a centering and connecting effect in the body.

3. As you may suspect, living the Concepts is not always easy. Usui himself, according to his Japanese students, found it challenging sometimes. In the words of Andrew Bowling, "He [Usui] could get righteously angry and quite impatient, particularly with people who wanted results but were not prepared to work for them." (See article at www.threshold.ca/Andrew-Bowling/Usui.html.)

4. In *O-Sensei: A View of Mikao Usui.*

5. Received by me through email.

6. Where she got this story I don't know. It certainly doesn't fit with the Gakkai version of history, which has Usui discovering his Reiki system

only four years before his passing. This in itself—as well as the fact that Takata's version had Usui discovering Reiki in the mid-1800s—is a strong indication that she was ignorant of the Usui Gakkai altogether.

7. The subject of money has been a major challenge for me in this lifetime, and it seems to be so for many Reiki people. When I started giving Reiki treatments, I set a price on my time; that was how it was done by my teacher, and by the other Reiki people I knew. Then, after a while, the Reiki itself led me to give it freely (accepting whatever the recipient chose to give in return). I wanted never again to put a price tag on anything! I saw truly that the Universe is a flawless accountant; that sometimes people are not able to give, materially, a fair exchange, but that such people are often the most grateful for what they receive; and that, regardless of what we are given by a particular individual, the Universe as a whole will never short-change us.

It seemed to me that price tags were based on fear and lack of trust: fear of not being given enough, lack of trust in the nature of the Universe. One of the Reiki Precepts deals with exactly that: letting go of fear and worry, having faith. So, I took the price tags off not just the Reiki, but everything I was doing, and I kept simplifying my way of living to require less and less money. But, as I required less, I received even less yet. Eventually I had too little money for even the most minimal lifestyle that allowed me to do my work.

It seemed that, yes, the Universe was an impeccable accountant, but it did not necessarily exchange energy in the form we desired. It seemed that, if we needed a certain amount of exchange in the form of money, we might indeed have to resort to price tags. Reluctantly, I began requesting specific amounts of money for some things. I continued giving Reiki treatments and Reiju freely, but asked for a specific donation for certified initiation in each official degree of Reiki. And I started asking a small donation for my Reiki e-book trilogy, though the first book remained free. (In either case, the donation was not required if it constituted a hardship.)

At this writing, I'm not entirely happy with such a compromise. Being a "middle way" of sorts, maybe it is indeed the best course. Maybe it's just the extremist in me that yearns to abolish all price tags. But I can't help feeling that they really should not be needed; that, if I'm clinging to even a single price tag, I'm not fully trusting divine providence. It occurs to me that maybe the way to receive more Universal exchange in the form of money is by giving more in the form of money. My inclination has been to give what I had the most of: time, energy, attention, work, friendship, and love. Maybe the key to unlocking this mystery is the giving of what I have least of: money. It seems an idea worth exploring. Maybe I can report on that exploration in a later book....

Chapter 3

1. I've also gone through periods of not doing this, when I thought I was too busy to afford the time for Reiki. Then, coming back to the daily Reiki, I've felt (always!): *How could I have been so crazy, to get my priorities out of order?* It reminds me of the great Lakota holy man Fools Crow, who said that the more things he had to do, the *more* time he spent praying, before starting to do them!

2. These are the seven chakras of the classic Indian system. There are also countless other systems of identifying and working with chakras.

3. The concept of yin and yang originated, as far as we know, in ancient China. The prevalent story is that, initially, yin was related to areas of shade in a natural environment, and yang to areas of sunlight. And, eventually the concept was expanded to encompass all imaginable pairs of complementary opposites (night/day, female/male, cold/hot, etc.). Heaven came to be seen as Great Yang (generative, creative, active), and Earth as Great Yin (receptive, passive).

   But there is another story, which says that the earliest concept of yin and yang was more or less the opposite of this; that it originated with a man named Fu Xi (or Fu Hsi), who defined the expansiveness of sky (Heaven) as yin, and the contractive firmness of Earth as yang. Fu Xi is credited with creating the sixty-four hexagrams of the *I Ching*. And later, it is said, a ruler in the Zhou Dynasty (King Wen) got hold of Fu Xi's hexagrams and changed them—so that today's *I Ching* equates Heaven with Great Yang and Earth with Great Yin. (For much more on the subject, see http://macrobiotics.johreiki.net/Yin_and_Yang.php.)

These two conflicting perceptions have created much confusion about yin and yang. Traditional Chinese Medicine, for example, views yin as contractive, yang as expansive; and Macrobiotics says just the opposite. Teachers of Macrobiotics assert that it doesn't matter which system of yin and yang we use, as long as we're consistent and don't mix the two. But there are problems even with that. For example: Both Macrobiotics and Traditional Chinese Medicine see maleness as characteristically yang, and femaleness as characteristically yin—and yet their definitions of yin and yang are opposite each other!

After years of muddling through this yin-yang maze myself, I have only recently encountered a ray of light that actually makes sense of yin and yang, once and for all. The expansive-contractive mystery is solved immediately by the most rudimentary knowledge of kototama. The sounds of the words themselves tell us that yin is contractive and yang is expansive! Just to be clear on the pronunciation of the words: Yin rhymes with "green" (long-E sound); Yang rhymes with "song" (Ahhh sound). Seie Brigham, a Kototama Life Therapist (and long-time student of Nakazono-sensei), points this out in an article posted at www.macrobiotics.co.uk/masahilonakazono.htm.

4. I know, the Taoists are flipping their wigs at some of my correlations. Sorry, but this is *my intuitive Universe!*

5. I was taught to cover the eyes with the fingers of both hands parallel, pointing straight up, which also puts the forearms parallel, in front of the body. I've since adopted the fingers-crossing position, which is more comfortable to the arms and also has the added benefit of concentrating more Reiki on the Brow Chakra. (I borrowed it from the palming technique of Dr. William Bates, who borrowed it from a Yoga technique.)

6. At second level (Okuden) and third level (Shinpiden), students are given

kotodama (primal sounds) and symbols to help them recognize aspects of these energies in themselves. One can start feeling the nature of the energies directly, though, at first level (Shoden)—and, to some degree, even without Reiki empowerment—when practicing this self-treatment.

7. "Over the years it has become clear," Dave wrote in an email, "that you still need to 'do the work' but it is done from a place of deep mindfulness—such as is found in Chado (tea ceremony). We do not waste time and effort 'getting in the way' of ourselves so only the minimum amount of effort is used."

8. Twin Lakes: Lotus Press, 2001.

Chapter 4

1. A translation of the Healing Guide (thanks to Rick Rivard) can be found at www.threshold.ca/reiki/Usui_Reiki_Hikkei.html. Another translation appears, in two parts, in *The Original Reiki Handbook of Dr. Mikao Usui* by Petter (Twin Lakes: Lotus Press, 1999) and *Reiki: The Legacy of Dr. Usui* (Twin Lakes: Lotus Press, 1999).

2. Taggart King points out that the Healing Guide is nearly identical to one published under Hayashi's name; also, that the whole idea of such a meticulous, recipe-book approach seems much more suited to Hayashi's disciplined medical and military style. We know that Hayashi devoted his own practice of Reiki to developing exactly this kind of system, correlating particular hand positions and physical symptoms. Also, both Andrew Bowling and Dave King have said that Dr. Hayashi created such a Guide, at Usui's request, in 1925.

3. When I learned Hatsurei-ho (see next section of this chapter), from Mr. Doi, this part of the exercise was done while breathing out through the mouth, whispering the sound of "Haaaa," almost like a sigh. This is called *hado* breathing. You will see later, in the section on kotodama, that this sound has the effect of "expanding the light of life."

4. When I learned Hatsurei-ho, from Mr. Doi, this part of the exercise (5–6 and 7) was done with arm extended and palm facing down or slightly to

the outside, and brushing the other hand the entire length of the extended arm, and beyond the fingertips.

5. See "The Gakkai's Okuden" in Chapter 6 for more details.

6. Mikoto Masahilo Nakazono, *The Source of the Present Civilization* (Santa Fe: Kototama Books, 1994), p. 5.

7. Mikoto Masahilo Nakazono, *Inochi—The Book of Life* (Santa Fe: Kototama Institute, 1984), pp. 1, 2, 6.

[8.] Nakazono defined "a priori" as: "the world of non-manifested life rhythms. In human expression, that which can be grasped by the spiritual senses." Mikoto Masahilo Nakazono, *The Source of the Present Civilization* (Santa Fe: Kototama Books, 1994), p. 239.

[9.] Nakazono defined "a posteriori" as: "the world of manifested life rhythms. In human expression, that which can be grasped by the physical senses." Ibid.

10. Ibid., p. 7.

11. *Inochi—The Book of Life*, p. 6. (See Note 7 above.)

12. The attention here is on the *letting go*.

13. "Source-dimension" is my name for what I feel is a non-physical, invisible dimension—something like an infinitesimally small Black Hole—within every wave-particle of physical matter. I feel it is the welling-up and overflowing of Source energy, in its countless forms, through this Source-dimension, that we perceive as manifested Life.

Chapter 5

[1.] Some people have translated this to mean the founding of the Usui Gakkai. See Note 10, Chapter 1, for more information.

2. Walter Lübeck describes these in more detail, in *The Spirit of Reiki* (Twin Lakes: Lotus Press, 2001).

3. Michio Kushi, *Macrobiotic Home Remedies* (New York: Japan Publications, Inc., 1985), p. 34.

I found this quotation interesting in that Kushi had equated Reiki with yin and yang. My own feeling had been that yin and yang arose at the level of Jiki (magnetism, polarity), and that Reiki, located just above that level, was indeed, as Walter Lübeck describes, the mysterious connector between the spiritual and physical realms. My feeling when experiencing Reiki has always been one of being suddenly connected to my true Self, to my Source. I believe that's what Reiki does for us, whether applied as a "treatment" or as an "empowerment/attunement." It feels to me like an "extension cord" connecting me to the Source.

However, Reiki teacher Mike Fuchs pointed out to me that yin and yang can never really be separated, that yin and yang together make up the indivisible reality of tai-chi—and that is what Kushi is referring to here, with the words "yin and yang." "Also," he says, "it is generally regarded that the energy/force depicted by the tai chi symbol is identical to the force/energy which is called either 'tao' or 'dao.' So, tai chi and dao are the same, just named differently...." If this is the case, then "reiki" and "dao" are also just two different words for the same thing: that indivisible, life force at the first level of manifestation, which brings about the dynamic balance of ever-changing energies in all things.

4. See www.threshold.ca/reiki/Highest_Ki.html for more from Rick Rivard. This report of Rivard's brings to mind the first time I received Johrei energy, and my feeling that it was more powerful than Reiki. But later I came to realize it had felt more powerful simply because it was a new energy to me. Once I got accustomed to it, I felt it less strongly—though it was (and is) somehow different than Reiki.

5. Copyright © 2002 Dave King; reprinted by permission. This and more can be seen at www.threshold.ca/reiki/Usui-Gainen.html.

6. I've had email contact with Taggart King since 2001, when he first sent me one of his Reiki manuals incorporating information from Chris Marsh. He later sent other manuals, updated as more was learned. The information presented here came from one of those.

7. Both books published by DeVorss & Company, Camarillo, California. Some writers have claimed that Max misinterpreted the ancient teachings. The word *aumakua,* for instance, which Max said referred to the "High Self,"

others have translated as "ghost of your ancestors." According to them, the aumakua is an ancestral spirit who agrees to come back to Earth and help us with advice and protection—*a concept seemingly identical with Tatsumi's belief about Usui's use of the word Reiki!* In any case, "ghost of your ancestors" is clearly the exoteric meaning of aumakua; Max believed "High Self" to be the esoteric meaning, which he had arrived at by deep and careful study of the many-layered Hawai'ian language. Considering that the whole realm of Huna is of things that are secret or hidden, it hardly makes sense that the exoteric, everyday meanings of words would be the ones involved. I feel that Max's interpretation is indeed correct.

8. *The Secret Science At Work,* p. 12.

Chapter 6

1. These descriptions are from one of Taggart's training manuals.
[2.] Also known as the five transformations or five energies—Water, Tree, Fire, Earth, Metal—this is an ancient Taoist concept.
3. *Lésé Majesté* is a French expression (literally, "injured majesty") referring to a perceived offense against a sovereign power or its ruler.

Chapter 7

[1.] Hawayo Takata was a minister in the Spiritualist Church.
[2.] All these quotations are from email correspondence with Dave.
[3.] Dave says: "The possible association of SUN/MOON/EARTH to the Amida Sanzon was not presented to me by any of my **Usui-Do** teachers. Mochizuki (who was teaching the 'mother' of TJR [Traditional Japanese Reiki], not Usui-Do) had given me photocopies of a book in Japanese that explained the Amida-Seishi-Kannon connections."
4. Mr. Rand presents his case, and pictures of the Kurama-Kokyo symbols, at www.reiki.org/reikinews/rootsreiki.html.
5. Again, in email correspondence.
6. This is from one of Taggart's manuals.
7. Again, this is from email correspondence.

8. In fact, there are different versions or understandings of kotodama/koto-tama in general (and my own study of them has barely begun). Kototama as used by Morihei Ueshiba were inspired by Onisaburo Deguchi's under-standing of kototama (Deguchi helped to develop the Omoto Kyo reli-gion); and within Aikido itself, some teach a system of fifty kototama and others teach seventy-five. Taggart King (in one of his manuals) asserts that Usui used "classical" kotodama, "not any new interpretation that may have come through Omoto-kyo. . . ."

9. Andy learned the kotodama from Chris Marsh, and was teaching them in workshops, with Chris, for some time.

10. For examples of both, see the section on kototama in "An Energy Exer-cise of My Own" (Chapter 4).

11. From *Inochi—The Book of Life,* p. 117.

[12.] "Kana: Word of God . . . True human language." Definition from Mikoto Masahilo Nakazono, *The Source of the Present Civilization* (Santa Fe: Kototama Books, 1994), p. 240.

Chapter 8

1. Dave King, email correspondence, 2002–2005.

2. All these quotes are from Volume One of *Mokichi Okada, The Light from the East,* compiled by The Church of World Messianity, *Sekai Kyusei Kyo* (Atami, Japan: MOA Productions, 1986).

3. See www.oomoto.or.jp/.

Chapter 9

1. The idea of "higher empowerments" is intriguing to me—but also it brings to mind something my Reiki friend Barb Emerson used to say: "Once you're connected to the Source of everything, how much *more* connected can you get??"

2. These quotes are from the manuals of Taggart King.

3. In fact, according to Dave King, "Dai Ko Myo!" is used commonly as an exclamation in China—something like "Good God!" or "I get it now!"

4. Before the Reiju, I also like to do the breathing exercise, with Reiki Concepts, described in Chapter 4 ("An Energy Exercise of My Own").

5. One of my students once reported perceiving the same Reiju twice! He was in England, I was in Hawai'i, and we had agreed to do Reiju at 8 p.m. GMT. I started doing my part an hour earlier—stipulating that the Reiju be perceived at 8:00, of course—and the student later told me that he had been working at his computer at 7:00 when he suddenly got a very strong mental message, "Reiju now!" and began feeling the energy. It continued for some time, then started again at 8:00!

Chapter 10

1. Rather than treating Metal as a separate entity, I include it in Earth. The Taoists, similarly, relate Metal to the Earth's minerals and the force of gravity. At the same time, they also relate Metal to the lungs and the element of Air!

2. "Steep Uphill Climb to 2012: Messages from the Mayan Milieu" © 2002 Steven McFadden. Reprinted by permission. The whole article can be seen at www.chiron-communications.com/communique%207-10.html.

3. These three quotes are from Mikoto Masahilo Nakazono, *The Source of the Present Civilization* (Santa Fe: Kototama Books, 1994), pp. 238–239. And, by the way, I can't help noticing that the three elements he describes are (1) "physical," (2) "spiritual," and (3) "complete"—sounding so very similar to Usui's "Earth," "Heaven," and "Oneness"!

4. *Ibid.,* p. 201.

5. My descriptions of these are compiled from various Web sources and *The Biology of Belief,* a book by Dr. Bruce Lipton (Santa Rosa: Mountain of Love/Elite Books, 2005). Dr. Lipton credits his descriptions of these brain states to Dr. Rima Laibow, in *Introduction to Quantitative EEG and Neurofeedback,* by James R. Evans and Andrew Abarbanel (Academic Press, 1999).

6. Idaho Falls: Rolling Thunder Publishing, 2006.

7. I don't know why, but it felt imperative to separate each individual syllable of certain words in this!

8. If you have a relatively short list, you may prefer to identify each individual separately. In any case, when I add someone new, I like to do a separate Reiju with that person alone, the first time (just to be sure a strong connection is made).

Chapter 11

1. Johrei Fellowship is the American counterpart of Sekai Kyusei Kyo ("Church of World Messianity") in Japan, and is officially (legally) a religion. For more information, see www.johrei.com.

2. The familiar "White Light" calligraphy was done by Okada's widow and was used after his passing. In recent years, some Johrei Centers in North America began using instead a calligraphy of Ko Myo, done by Okada himself.

3. *Sama* is a term of reverence. Ever since the Kannon Society, Okada has been referred to by his followers as Meishu-sama. (In a similar way, some of Usui's students have referred to him as Usui-sama.) And, thanks to the mysteries of the Japanese language, "Meishu" ("Spiritual Leader") is also translated as "Lord of Light"!

4. Two articles, written by Okada on these subjects, may be of interest. An English translation of one ("My Light"—May 25, 1952) can be seen at www.jinsai.org/english/meishu_sama/history/histjins06.php . . . and the other ("Johrei and the Three-element Composition of the Internal Organs"—August 6, 1949) at www.jinsai.org/english/teachings/johrei/teachjoh02.php.

Chapter 12

1. Frederick Bailes, *Your Mind Can Heal You* (Camarillo, CA: DeVorss & Company, 1941).

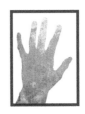

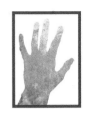

About the Author

DON BECKETT, born and raised in Colorado, has also lived in Hawai'i, Oregon, Utah, Mexico, and Bali. He currently calls Mesa, Arizona, home. He has been practicing Reiki since 1991 and has initiated others since 1999. He has also practiced various kinds of formal meditation for more than twenty-five years and is a member of the Johrei Fellowship. Beckett's Web site johreiki.net attracts thousands of teachers and students of Reiki from all over the world.